Praise for The 8-Hour Sleep Paradox

This is one of the most important books on health I have read in a while. As a doctor, author, and lecturer who even gives talks on sleep, I thought I had a good understanding of the subject, but Dr. Burhenne adds a dimension that no other book so clearly addresses. The book has changed the way I view my own sleep and will forever change the way I educate my patients and audience about this critical subject. I guarantee you or someone close to you will benefit profoundly from this information. An absolute must-read.

Ronesh Sinha, MD, author of The South Asian Health Solution

Dr. Mark Burhenne is a pioneering voice in the prevention and treatment of sleep apnea. This guide presents his straightforward, action-oriented plan for healing by measuring, treating, and verifying your sleep quality for a lifetime of healing, deep sleep. This book revolutionizes the way we understand and treat our sleep. I highly recommend it!

Mark Hyman, MD, #1 New York Times bestselling author of The Blood Sugar Solution and Director of th Cleveland Clinic Center for Functional Medicine

There are few iron laws of the universe, but here's one: if you want to be happier, healthier, and more productive, you need to get enough sleep. *The 8-Hour Sleep Paradox* will help you improve the quality of your sleep, so you'll feel more alive than ever.

Gretchen Rubin, #1 New York Times bestselling author of Better Than Before, The Happiness Project and Happier at Home.

If you want to boost your brainpower, memory, energy, and mood, as well wake up every morning happy and in the driver's seat of your life, Dr. Burhenne is your guide. In this groundbreaking book, he shows us how every one of us is susceptible to sleep breathing interruptions and what to do to optimize this breathing for efficient, optimal, and healing sleep every night of our lives.

Frank Lipman, MD, New York Times bestselling author of The New Health Rules, founder and director of Eleven-Eleven Wellness in New York City and creator of Be Well by Dr. Frank Lipman

When I work with my clients and when I lecture to medical professionals and CEOs alike, I tell them that if they do not take anything home with them that day, to take home this message: Your body needs fuel and that comes in the form of the quality foods you eat and the quality sleep you get. I can't stress enough how important this book is for people to read as it will help you better understand why you need quality sleep, what the pitfalls or correctable problems may be that are preventing you from getting it, and what you can do about it. I highly recommend you read The 8-Hour Sleep Paradox and get yourself feeling better than you thought possible.

Eva Selhub, MD, Harvard Medical School Lecturer in Medicine and author of Your Health Destiny and The Love Response

Getting good sleep is one of the most precious things we can do for our long-term health. When patients come to me unable to lose weight, get their blood pressure under control, fix their sugar cravings, or get over daytime fatigue, the first thing I look to is their sleep. And so often, it turns out that, sure enough, there is a sleep disorder at the root of their problem. In this book, Dr. Burhenne will help you to find out whether you have a sleep disorder that is preventing you from having the health you deserve and living the life you want. When looking for the root causes of your chronic health problems, make sure to look in this important resource!

Aviva Romm, MD, award-winning author, creator of WomanWise and founder of the Yale Integrative Medicine program

The 8-Hour Sleep Paradox

How We Are Sleeping Our Way to Fatigue, Disease, and Unhappiness

Mark Burhenne, DDS

Mark Burhenne, DDS

Sunnyvale, CA 94087

© 2015 Dr. Mark Burhenne

Table of Contents

For my mom and dad

Chapter 1:
Why Is a Dentist
Writing About Sleep?

It was Friday morning, and I was being whacked in the face with three pillows. I blinked awake and looked around. Each of the pillows belonged to one of my three daughters. It was 2006, and the entire family had slept in the same hotel room.

"Dad! You were so noisy last night, we could barely sleep!" my daughters complained. "It sounded like there was a freight train in the room!"

Being woken via pillow whacking had done nothing for my humor, and I sarcastically replied that there were, in fact, train tracks outside the window—so maybe what they'd heard really had been a freight train. They weren't impressed.

Despite my early morning sarcasm, I began to think about the snoring more seriously. Weren't people who snored overweight and unhealthy? At breakfast that morning, my wife began chatting with another hotel guest. He told me I should get checked for sleep apnea.

That seemed reasonable, so off I went to my primary care physician. I was referred to an ENT (ear, nose, and throat doctor), who scheduled me for a home sleep study. The night of the test, a man came by the house to "hook me up." I had things glued to my face and chest. As I tried to fall asleep, I noticed I was hooked up to a computer with flashing LED lights and a noisy hard drive.

Feeling very clever, I made some modifications. I wrapped the computer in a towel and put the whole bundle under the bed. Then I jumped into bed and had what I thought was my normal, restful night of sleep.

Six weeks later, I got the results from my ENT. "You passed the test!" he said. "You're fine." He sent me home with a diagnosis of mild sleep apnea and, since it was only mild, no suggestions for any kind of treatment. Years later, I would realize the consequences of not treating even "mild" sleep apnea.

The question remained: if I was fine, then where had the snoring been coming from, that night in the hotel? It couldn't have been my wife, could it?

My wife, Roseann, is one of the most health-conscious people I know. She regularly wakes up at 5:30 a.m. for a Pilates or spin class. She has cut gluten and grains from her diet. She meditates daily and never forgets to take her vitamins. She doesn't have a sweet tooth like I do. She's petite and thin. For a while, we jokingly referred to her as the "flax fairy," because she'd walk past our breakfast plates and squirt flax oil on top.

There's no way it could have been Roseann snoring that night. She was the picture of health. But then I thought about it a bit more. Even though she was living well, she had bouts of depression. She'd been diagnosed with a heart condition. Her blood pressure and cholesterol were on the rise for no apparent reason. She'd had an early menopause that baffled us. She was one of those people who was *always* sick. She had recurrent sinus infections. She had intolerances to many different foods. In her forties, we had to block off weekend afternoons so she could nap. She was working hard, so this didn't concern either of us. Every morning, she woke up absolutely exhausted, but wasn't that just a part of being in your forties? She relied on daily exercise to give her energy. She couldn't stay awake through movies. Could it have been her immune system, heart, and mental health were suffering because her sleep was suffering?

The mystery was solved as soon as Roseann's sleep study results came back: her breathing was being interrupted over 34.5 times per *hour* each night.

Like unplugging your hard drive during a backup, interruptions in the brain's sleep cycles have serious consequences. After each interruption, the brain doesn't pick up where it left off—it starts over. The brain cannot do its essential repair work when it is repeatedly interrupted. Roseann had been suffering from these breathing interruptions every night for years, decades—maybe even her whole life.

The day she got her diagnosis was the day I began learning everything I could about sleep breathing. My research led me so far into the world of sleep, I became determined to share what I'd learned with my patients. I began the process of becoming certified in dental sleep medicine, an area where dentists are working together with sleep physicians to screen for and treat sleep breathing conditions so they're caught and corrected earlier. I began screening my patients for the signs of sleep conditions that show up in the mouth, referring them to sleep specialists, and creating mouthguard-style devices for them to wear during sleep—devices that moved their jaws forward to help them sleep better.

Now, nearly thirty years after graduating from dental school, after living through my wife's sleep apnea diagnosis and my own, and after treating my patients with sleep breathing disorders, I'm able to connect the dots. This is what I learned: sleep determines our destinies.

We had no idea Roseann wasn't sleeping well. I certainly didn't notice anything wrong with her breathing—but then again, I'd been asleep. I'd slept through her suffering not once, but during hundreds of breathing interruptions every night. In hindsight, I can see that there were plenty of warning signs—just not ones we knew about back then. We'll discuss those in this book.

How Your Teeth Affect Your Sleep

When you think of your mouth, you probably picture your teeth and your gums. But this is just scratching the surface of how our teeth impact the health of the rest of our bodies.

The placement of teeth in your mouth affects the placement of everything else, including your jaw, tongue, facial muscles, and throat. When teeth are crowded, the rest of your craniofacial development is crowded. Among other things, crowded teeth reduce the amount of space you have at the back of your throat— the amount of space you can use to breathe. Everything in your mouth determines how well you breathe at night, and therefore how well you sleep.

I'll explain more about the breathing and sleep connection throughout this book. While it may seem inconceivable that you could have difficulty breathing at night, you'll soon understand how the modern diet and lifestyle make interrupted breathing during sleep so common that it has become an epidemic.

The Sleep Ability Quiz

These questions are designed to give you some insight into your sleep ability—that is, your body's ability to breathe easily even as it becomes paralyzed in the deepest stages of sleep.

If you answer yes to any of these questions, your sleep ability may be suffering.

✓ Do you have a family history of sleep apnea, sleep-disordered breathing, or other sleep-related issues or conditions?

✓ Do you prefer one side when sleeping?

✓ Do you have a scalloped or fissured tongue? (Little teeth marks on the side of the tongue or a groove running down the middle of the tongue.)

✓ Do you have acid erosion on your upper teeth?

✓ Do you grind or clench your teeth?

✓ Do you have pain, clicking, or popping in your jaw?

✓ Do you crave carbohydrates or caffeine for energy?

✓ Do you fall asleep right when you hit the pillow? Anything less than 10 or 15 minutes might mean you're sleep deprived.

✓ Do you have trouble falling asleep?

✓ Are you hyperactive or high energy?

✓ Do you crave naps?

✓ Did you suck your thumb as a child?

✓ Does your sleep partner tell you that you snore?

✓ Do you wake up unrefreshed?

✓ Do you get sleepy and tired during the day?

✓ Do you need several alarms to wake up in the morning to get to work or school?

✓ Do you wake up with a dry mouth?

✓ Do you wake up with a headache or neck ache?

✓ Do you have high blood pressure or very low blood pressure?

✓ Do you have a steep jawline (called a steep mandibular plane)?

✓ Do you have a receding chin?

✓ Do you have a tight band of tissue that tethers the bottom of the tip of your tongue to the floor of your mouth? (tongue-tie, or lingual frenulum)

✓ Do you have GERD (gastroesophageal reflux disease)?

✓ Do you have frequent nosebleeds?

✓ Have you ever had an injury to your nose?

✓ Do you have frequent trouble with sinusitis?

✓ Do you have pressure in your sinuses or nasal congestion?

✓ Do you have gout?

Sleep Myths That Are Killing Us

Myth 1: If You're Not Snoring, You're Fine

If you're already snoring, your sleep issues were not caught early enough. Our healthcare system only looks for symptoms of late-stage illness and disease, rather than trying to intervene early. We are failing to catch and treat sleep breathing issues early on. I've seen patients whose interrupted sleep breathing wasn't treated simply because they were young, healthy, and thin.

Myth 2: I Don't Have Sleep Apnea, So I'm Fine

I'll always regret not pushing my doctor to treat me after he told me I was "fine" because I had "only" mild sleep apnea. I wasn't fine. But in any case, sleep apnea represents a tiny fraction of the wide spectrum of sleep disorders. By stopping at ruling out sleep apnea, we fail to treat millions of people who have suboptimal sleep for some other reason.

Myth 3: Weight Loss Is Necessary to Improve Sleep Quality

While weight loss does help significantly, losing weight is a massive lifestyle change that can take years. Opening up your airway so you breathe better at night improves sleep quality, which can actually *accelerate* weight loss.

Myth 4: Children Are the Best Sleepers

You've heard the expression "sleeping like a baby," but children have several unique challenges when it comes to breathing during sleep. Growing bodies often haven't caught up with large tonsils and tongues, which can cause breathing difficulty at night. Things like diet, use of sippy cups, length of breastfeeding, and allergies all impact how a child's face, mouth, teeth, jaw, and airway develop—setting the stage for what the child's sleep quality will be as he or she grows older.

Myth 5: People With Sleep Disorders Have to Sleep With a Machine

First of all, I'd like to get this out there: sleep machines aren't scary. They aren't difficult to use, they aren't painful, and they shouldn't be feared. But if for whatever reason a CPAP or APAP machine isn't right for you—don't worry! There are other options.

Myth 6: It's Adorable When My Child/Partner/Friend Snores

I imagine a world where, one day, we consider snoring to be as serious as smoking. Snoring is never normal, never cute, and always a red flag for poor sleep.

Myth 7: Sleep Problems Can Be Cured Using Sleep Hacks

There are lots of sleep hacks out there for improving sleep quality—such as minimizing blue light before bed or not drinking caffeine after 2 p.m. Sleep hygiene is important, but in comparison to sleep breathing, they're icing on the cake. Optimizing your sleep breathing isn't just the best bang for your buck—it trumps so many of these sleep hacks because you're too knocked out in deep sleep to notice the temperature of the room.

After getting treated, Roseann now breathes so well that she doesn't have a single interruption in her breathing at night. Not one. Her sleep study came back with a big fat zero on the charts. Improved sleep has made big changes in Roseann's life. We get to have regular date nights again, and she can stay awake through movies. Her blood pressure and cholesterol went back down to healthy levels soon after treatment. Most of all, she's felt much greater fulfillment and satisfaction with life. She used to live life on a treadmill—always running to the next thing, in a brain fog that she'd assumed was just a part of working hard. Now, after a decade of getting the best sleep of her life, she has never felt sharper, better, or more alive.

Understanding the Epidemic

Sleep is that golden chain that ties health and our bodies together.
—Thomas Dekker

Fundamental to the mission of the National Institutes of
Health (NIH) to foster health research is the solemn obligation
to be absolutely certain that American citizens actually receive
the benefits derived from this research. I am sorry to say that in
the area of sleep deprivation and sleep disorders, knowledge
transfer has largely failed.
—Dr. William C. Dement, MD, PhD,
in a statement to Congress March 26, 1998

Imagine you're in bed. Your eyes slowly open, and you realize it's morning. It's still several minutes before the alarm is set to go off. You feel peaceful and rested. You slowly begin to peel out of bed, and every muscle in your body is coming out of a state of deep relaxation. You feel sharp, fully awake, clear-headed, and ready to take on the day. All of this describes the perfect night's sleep—and, no, I'm not talking about getting your eight hours, because the number of hours you get is of no consequence if you're not breathing properly.

Sleep-disordered breathing is a condition that describes the entire spectrum of sleep breathing abnormalities. The sleep-disordered breathing spectrum ranges from more mild breathing difficulties—caused by things like a stuffy nose or sleeping on your back—to the more severe conditions—like snoring and sleep apnea.

Living in the modern world has changed how all of us sleep. Beginning from birth, we're exposed to things like pacifiers, bottles, and sippy cups that change the development of our face, jaw, tongue, teeth—ultimately making the tiny space at the back of our throat that we rely on to breathe (i.e. the airway) narrower and narrower. Then, as adults who grow up with small airways, we don't know we have a problem because we've never known what a true night of sleep feels like.

As a result, most of us are operating at suboptimal levels all the time. And it's not just short-term sleepiness we have to worry about; sleep-disordered breathing is an insidious inflammatory disease that affects every system in the body. It's associated with the biggest killers in the Western world: high blood pressure, strokes, cancer, heart disease, Alzheimer's, diabetes, and even depression.[1] When sleep breathing is disturbed, so is the essential repair work our bodies do each night to keep us happy, sharp, and disease-free.

Sleep-disordered breathing is insidious because the effects are so gradual that we don't notice them, and healthcare practitioners are not trained on how to recognize the symptoms in their earliest stages. Elementary schools screen children for vision, hearing, and even scoliosis, but not sleep disorders. People who suffer from chronic fatigue, headaches, exhaustion, irritable bowel syndrome,

---

1   Sarah Boseley, "Depression is the west's second biggest killer," The Guardian, 1999, *http://www.theguardian.com/uk/1999/may/12/sarahboseley.*

or unexplained weight gain are puzzled as to the cause of their ailments, and so are their doctors—and yet sleep breathing is rarely considered as a root cause.

We're concerned with how *much* sleep we're getting or sleep hygiene factors such as darkening the room or reducing blue light before bedtime, but none of those things matter if your sleep breathing is being interrupted.

Sleep-Disordered Breathing: More Common Than You May Think

➡ About 42 million American adults have sleep-disordered breathing,[2] up to 90% of which are undiagnosed.

➡ One in five adults has mild obstructive sleep apnea.[3]

➡ One in fifteen adults has moderate to severe obstructive sleep apnea.

➡ 80-90% of people with diabetes have obstructive sleep apnea.

➡ 50-95% of people who have had a stroke also have obstructive sleep apnea.

➡ 20-35% of people with heart failure have obstructive sleep apnea.

➡ Risk of nighttime arrhythmias increases up to four times in people with severe sleep disordered breathing.[4]

➡ People with moderate to severe sleep apnea have an up to 15-fold increase of being involved in a traffic accident.[5]

---

2   Young et al. *New Engl J Med*, 1993.

3   Young et al. *J Am Med Assoc*, 2004.

4   Reena Mehra, Emelia J. Benjamin, Eyal Shahar, Daniel J. Gottlieb, Rawan Nawabit, H. Lester Kirchner, Jayakumar Sahadevan, and Susan Redline, "Association of Nocturnal Arrhythmias with Sleep-disordered Breathing: The Sleep Heart Health Study," *American Journal of Respiratory and Critical Care Medicine* 173, no. 8 (2006): 910-916, doi: 10.1164/rccm.200509-1442OC.

5   Horstmann et al. *Sleep* (2000).

Sleep-Disordered Breathing and Mental Health

This isn't about just being sleepy; sleep disorders affect our judgment, emotional capacity, creativity, and just about every cognitive process. Scientists have found there's a strong link between anxiety and depression and sleep disorders. Yet, when someone is diagnosed with anxiety or depression, they're rarely offered a sleep study.

Problems Associated with Obstructive Sleep Apnea

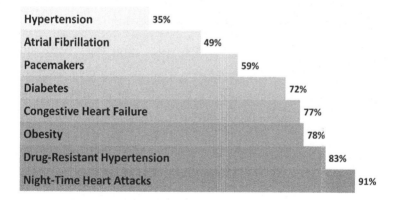

Hypertension	35%
Atrial Fibrillation	49%
Pacemakers	59%
Diabetes	72%
Congestive Heart Failure	77%
Obesity	78%
Drug-Resistant Hypertension	83%
Night-Time Heart Attacks	91%

A Public Health Crisis

The sleep-disordered breathing crisis is making us exhausted, sick, unhappy, and stupid. Sleep-disordered breathing now rivals obesity and smoking as our greatest public health crisis. I believe sleep-disordered breathing will come to be known as one of the biggest global health epidemics of our time. Today, the National Sleep Foundation estimates that two-thirds of all Americans have some sort of sleep disorder. Insufficient sleep is a public health epidemic[6], and yet it's only been in recent years that public health organizations such as the CDC have started making recommendations.

- ✓ Sleep deprivation impairs our brains as much as alcohol.

- ✓ 23% of adults have fallen asleep while driving.

- ✓ Up to one third of fatal crashes involve a driver who is sleep deprived, according to the Centers for Disease Control and Prevention (CDC).[7]

- ✓ Polls conducted by the National Sleep Foundation found that 60% of drivers have driven while sleepy.[8]

Driving while sleep deprived is risky, sometimes fatal, and more than half of us are doing it. It's not just our own sleep we have to worry about anymore—it's the sleep of the driver in the car next to us, our children's bus driver, or our airplane pilot.

---

6   "Insufficient Sleep Is a Public Health Problem," *Centers for Disease Control and Prevention*, 2015, *http://www.cdc.gov/features/dssleep/*.

7   "Morbidity and Mortality Weekly Report (MMWR): Drowsy Driving—19 States and the District of Columbia, 2009-2010," *Centers for Disease Control and Prevention*, 2013, *http://www.cdc.gov/mmwr/preview/mmwrhtml/mm6151a1.htm?s_cid=mm6151a1_w*.

8   "Summary of Findings: 2005 Sleep in America Poll," *National Sleep Foundation*, 2005, *http://sleepfoundation.org/sites/default/files/2005_summary_of_findings.pdf*.

Economic Costs of Sleep Deprivation:

✓ The total economic cost of sleepiness is $43-56 billion.[9]

✓ Untreated sleep apnea may cause $3.4 billion in additional medical costs in the U.S.[10]

✓ Prior to sleep apnea diagnosis, patients utilized 23-50% more medical resources.[11]

Sleep and Denial

Here's perhaps the most dangerous part: we are in denial about how we're sleeping—and I include myself in that statement. My patients who are entrepreneurs, students, surgeons, pilots, and bus drivers all tell me the same thing: "I don't have time to get a sleep study." But sleep-disordered breathing reduces our productivity and even earnings. In fact, the biochemical restoration that the brain and body go through during sleep is so powerful that brushing off sleep is akin to saying, "Yep, I'm okay with a little brain damage every day for the rest of my life."

Skipping sleep has become a badge of honor that proves total dedication to work. Leaders, politicians, and coworkers brag that they'll stay up late and get up early to work hard and get the job done. But true dedication isn't skimping on sleep—it's becoming the most efficient sleeper you can to optimize performance, and this means taking your sleep ability seriously.

---

9   Leger et al. *Sleep*, 1994.

10   Vishesh Kapur, David K. Blough, Robert E. Sandblom, Richard Hert, James B. de Maine, Sean D. Sullivan, Bruce M. Psaty, "The Medical Cost Of Undiagnosed Sleep Apnea," Sleep 22, no. 6 (2015), *http://www.journalsleep.org/ViewAbstract.aspx?pid=24161.*

11   Smith et al. *Chest* (2002).

Even if you're able to barrel through the short-term effects of sleep deprivation, there's no escape from the long-term effects. As the damage accumulates, the immune system is weakened[12] and you increase your risk of multiple types of cancer[13]. The body[14] becomes more susceptible to metabolic and endocrine issues, raising the risk of heart disease and diabetes. You accelerate cognitive decline, increasing your chances of dementia and Alzheimer's.[15] People with untreated sleep disorders have a 20% shorter life expectancy.

That is why I cringe every time I come across another viral video of a "hilarious snoring woman who sounds like a plane" or an "adorable" snoring baby. Sleep-disordered breathing is so common now that we don't even know what normal, healthy sleep breathing looks like.

---

12   David F. Dinges, Steven D. Douglas, Steffi Hamarman, Line Zaugg, and Shiv Kapoor. "Sleep deprivation and human immune function." *Advances in Neuroimmunology* 5, no. 2 (1995): 97–110, doi:10.1016/0960-5428(95)00002-J.

13   Kirsten C.G. Van Dycke, Wendy Rodenburg, Conny T.M. van Oostrom, Linda W.M. van Kerkhof, Jeroen L.A. Pennings, Till Roenneberg, Harry van Steeg, Gijsbertus T.J. van der Horst. "Chronically Alternating Light Cycles Increase Breast Cancer Risk in Mice." *Current Biology* 25, no. 14 (2015): 1932–1937, DOI: *http://dx.doi.org/10.1016/j. cub.2015.06.012.*

14   Sandra Sephtona, David Spiegel. "Circadian disruption in cancer: a neuroendocrine-immune pathway from stress to disease?" *ScienceDirect 17*, no. 5 (2003): 321–328, doi: 10.1016/S0889-1591(03)00078-3.

15   Jon Hamilton writes,
      Lack of sleep "not only increases the risk of errors and accidents, it also has adverse effects on the body and brain," according to Charles Czeisler, chief of the division of sleep and circadian disorders at Brigham and Women's Hospital in Boston.
      Research . . . has shown that a lack of sleep increases a person's risk for cardiovascular disease, diabetes, infections and maybe even Alzheimer's disease. Yet most sleep disorders go untreated.
      Jon Hamilton, "Snooze Alert: A Sleep Disorder May Be Harming Your Body And Brain," National Public Radio, 2015, *http://www.npr.org/sections/health-shots/2015/08/24/432764792/snooze-alert-a-sleep-disorder-may-be-harming-your-body-and-brain.*

Why the Healthiest Often Suffer Most with Sleep-Disordered Breathing

The people who suffer the most are perhaps the people who seem the healthiest. The younger and more symptom-free you are, the less likely your doctor is to suspect anything could be wrong with your sleep. I was one of these. I don't fit the profile that doctors look for, which is an overweight, middle-aged male with a thick neck who snores like a train. I was young, fit, and healthy. I never complained of fatigue. If I ever felt tired, I chalked it up to getting older or a really busy day. This disguised many of my symptoms. No doctor was going to prescribe an expensive sleep study to a young, fit male who had plenty of energy.

Some of the most common groups of people with undiagnosed sleep disorders are athletes, allergy sufferers, children with ADD/ADHD, petite women, and people who grind and clench their teeth. Their sleep disorders aren't caught because we aren't looking for the early-stage symptoms, and so they are falling through the cracks of the healthcare system.

The bottom line: even if you're perfectly healthy, you could be a ticking time bomb if you're not breathing well during sleep.

We are not healthy unless our sleep is healthy. Are you assuming your sleep is healthy because you feel like nothing's wrong? It's a lot to assume.

The Solution to Reverse the Sleep-Disordered Breathing Epidemic

Sleep is an exceptionally high-cost activity for our bodies to perform. Think about it: our bodies have to completely shut down for one third of each day. Earlier in our evolutionary history, that was a lot of time to spend vulnerable to attack and unable to defend ourselves. And yet this high cost and the amount of time our bodies demand we spend in sleep speaks to how important sleep is. Can you think of anything else you spend one third of your life doing? Even a 50-hour work week doesn't amount to that much. You could say that sleep is the most important job you have.

We age and we die of inflammatory diseases, meaning that the name of the game is to reduce inflammation in your body. The body naturally becomes inflamed as part of a healthy response to help us heal from injury and infection. But when inflammation is always present, it damages healthy tissue. Chronic inflammation speeds up the aging process and plays a key role in many ailments, including arthritis, heart disease, diabetes, fibromyalgia, osteoporosis, gingivitis, periodontitis, high blood pressure, stroke, obesity, asthma, dementia, and even some cancers. One of the largest contributors to chronic inflammation is sleep-disordered breathing. When you start breathing better at night, everything else falls into place—even cravings for inflammatory foods will be decreased. We can't control the size of our airway, which was determined by our childhood, but we *can* control how we breathe at night.

Millions of adults and children will be treated this year for depression, anxiety, heart conditions, weight gain, thyroid trouble, GERD (gastroesophageal reflux disease), and ADHD. They and their healthcare providers won't once stop to consider that these issues could be tied to an underlying cause: a sleep disorder.

As rates of disease, fatigue, and unhappiness all continue to skyrocket, teams of scientists are scrambling to find cures. But someone has to stand up and say the answer isn't another pharmaceutical drug—it's sleep—and our power to heal lies in optimizing our sleep ability so we can breathe and sleep as nature intended.

My solution: get screened early. Measure your sleep ability and treat your sleep so that you're getting your best night's sleep possible. Let the healing powers of sleep do the rest.

That is why I've written this book and why you're getting the perspective of a dentist who screens for sleep-disordered breathing every day. The signs of sleep-disordered breathing show up first in the mouth, jaw, and face, which is why the newest guidelines put forth by the American Academy of Sleep Medicine (AASM) and the American Academy of Dental Sleep Medicine (AADSM) have dentists on the frontlines, screening for sleep-disordered breathing at every six-month checkup.

I've helped thousands of my patients optimize their sleep breathing by using the approach outlined in this book, and, even after years of doing this, I'm still amazed by their incredible recoveries.

Getting Started

This book opened with a simple quiz to help assess your risk factors for sleep-disordered breathing. It was designed to get you out of denial and to be really honest with yourself about how well you're sleeping. Since many of us have allergies, small jaws, and large tongues, don't be surprised if you found yourself answering "yes" to many of the questions. Sleep-disordered breathing is common, but it's also very treatable, and what if it's the missing link to a better life you never knew you were missing?

In Chapter 2, I'll explain the latest scientific advances in our understanding of the airway-body biology. We'll discuss what sleep-disordered breathing is, what causes it, and the biology of how your sleep breathing affects every other system in your body.

In Chapters 3-6, you'll be walked through my three-step system to measure, treat, and verify your sleep ability in partnership with a sleep team.

The plan outlines:

✓ How to identify the underlying cause of your sleep breathing problems

✓ How to optimize your sleep breathing

✓ How to know which tests to get and when

✓ How to work with your doctor

✓ How to put together a sleep team that works together on your behalf

✓ How to verify you're getting healthy sleep for life

✓ What you should expect from every member of your sleep team: sleep specialist, dentist, myofunctional therapist, etc.

In Chapter 7, I'll show you how to get medical insurance coverage if you get your sleep-disordered breathing treated by your dentist.

Whether you are healthy now or have been suffering from sleep apnea for years, you can optimize your sleep breathing to become your brightest, happiest, most capable self.

My wife and I are in our mid-fifties, and we're entering our golden years in the best health of our lives. We have plenty of energy to backpack together for a week at a time. We easily keep up with our three adult daughters. I don't want to think about what might have happened to us had we never treated our sleep-disordered breathing.

What I want to pass on to you in this book is everything I've learned, not only as a sleep medicine dentist, but also as someone who has lived through treating my own sleep breathing. This book will help you shortcut much of what I, my family, and my patients have gone through in order to transform our sleep, our health, and our lives.

Chapter 2:
How We Sleep Is How We Live

A good laugh and a long sleep are the best cures in the doctor's book.

—*Irish Proverb*

As I write this book, I am overcome with the deep sadness of knowing that this information might have changed the fate of my father, who died in 1996 after his brain and body were ravaged by dementia and ALS at the age of 69. My father was once one of the most celebrated radiologists in the world.

He taught at Harvard, wrote textbooks, and developed the Burhenne technique[16] for removing gallstones. He led quite a life and, by all external measures, was an extremely fit and healthy man. He was a competitive downhill skier and accomplished mountaineer, and we summited several of North America's tallest mountains together. In short, he was hardly someone you would associate with breathing difficulties.

I've often wondered how such a healthy man could have deteriorated in such a spectacular way. Many chalk it up to genetics, but this simply doesn't fit with how modern diseases like ALS, cancer, and Alzheimer's continue to spike in the developed world despite our improved access to medicine and nutrition.

My father ate well, had a low body mass index (BMI), and was a tremendous athlete. But something, or multiple things, went very wrong and set off a chain of events in his body and brain. Looking back, I believe he wasn't able to stay in deep-stage sleep at night. Having been my dad's dentist, I now realize that the signs that he was suffering from a sleep breathing disorder were there in his mouth—they just weren't anything we learned about in dental school thirty years ago. If someone could have intervened early and helped him breathe better during sleep, he could have had a much longer life and greater health in his later years.

---

16   H. Joachim Burhenne, "Nonoperative Retained Biliary Tract Stone Extraction: A New Roentgenologic Technique," *American Journal of Roentgenology 117*, no. 2 (1973): 388-399, doi: 10.2214/ajr.117.2.388.

What does your mouth have to do with sleep? That's what we're going to explore in this chapter. We'll connect the dots between the chemical and biological changes that occur in the body during sleep and the surprising reason that breathing during sleep can be excruciatingly difficult.

Sleep Ability: The Most Important Health Stat You Don't Know

*It ain't what you don't know that gets you into trouble.
It's what you know for sure that just ain't so.*
—Mark Twain

Breathing is the single most important immediate physiological activity that we all must do to live. If you force your brain to choose between sleep and breathing, breathing will win every time.

Why would the brain have to choose between breathing and sleep? The reason is an anatomical problem: modern humans are developing with smaller jaws and smaller airways than humans centuries ago.

Imagine you live in a spacious apartment now, but are moving to a smaller apartment. When you move, the size of your furniture doesn't change. That means things are going to feel a lot tighter and more constricted inside your new, smaller apartment.

Our smaller jaws, thanks to the modern diet and lifestyle, are a lot like that smaller apartment. There's less room, but our tongue and voice box still take up the same amount of space.

When it comes to proper airway development, the cards are stacked against us: allergies, food sensitivities, chronic nasal congestion, and asthma all cause us to breathe through our mouths instead of our noses. As a result, we develop receding chins and weaker profiles, which leave less room for the airway.[17] Thanks to our diet of easy-to-chew foods beginning from infancy, our jaws aren't only smaller; they also don't grow down and out like they used to. This has devastating effects on the size of the airway.

In the dental office, we see the effects of this crowding because the teeth don't have enough room to come in straight. When children have to breathe through their mouths instead of noses, the tongue is no longer in the right position to keep teeth straight and act as nature's braces. But the real concern isn't crooked teeth—it's a small airway.

---

17   Patrick McKeown, "Mouth Breathing and Facial Development," *Buteyko Children*, accessed 09/2015, *http://www.buteykochildren.com/mouth_breathing_and_facial_development.php*. McKeown suggests (and describes) a simple method called the Buteyko Method to help children develop properly.

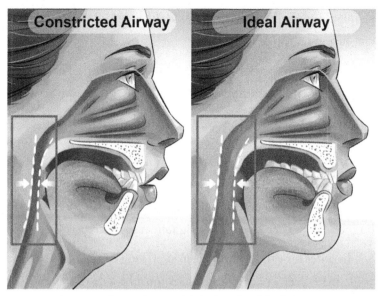

A comparison of a constricted and an ideal airway.

Despite our smaller airways, our breathing is automatic during our waking hours. As you read the words on this page, your airway is held open by the taut muscles in your neck and throat. Your tongue, also a muscle, is flat and pulled forward. Nothing is blocking vital oxygen from flowing in through your nose, over the back of your tongue, down your throat, and into your lungs, providing your bodily tissues with essential oxygen.

This picture changes drastically when we go to sleep. As we approach deep-stage sleep, the muscles that normally keep our airways propped open are turned off and go limp. The tongue, also a muscle, goes from toned and flat to a spread-out, floppy lump at the back of the throat, blocking the airway. In MRIs of people sleeping, the tongue in its flaccid state looks like a racquet ball sitting on top of the airway.

It's in deep sleep that the airway becomes too narrow to support effortless breathing. In extreme cases, the airway becomes so narrow that breathing stops completely. Every time this happens, the brain has to figure out a way to get you breathing again, at any cost. The brain stops what it's doing in deep sleep to tense up your muscles so they support the airway again. You don't have to wake up when this happens, but your brain does have to bounce out of deep sleep into a lighter stage of sleep.

In order for you to stay in deep sleep long enough to complete your entire sleep cycle, your muscles must be able to stay in their shut-off, completely relaxed state.

In healthy people, the airway stays open even when the muscles become paralyzed.[18] But for most of us, this isn't possible. Our airways have gotten smaller while everything else has stayed the same size, so we're left with bodies that aren't equipped to keep breathing while in deep-stage sleep.

It's not your breathing that suffers with these interruptions; it's your sleep. Each time the brain has to deal with a breathing interruption, it can't pick up where it left off—it has to start over. This means your body isn't able to fully complete stages of deep sleep. In extreme cases, your body may never even reach deep sleep.

---

18   The muscles are paralyzed, except for the heart, which continues to pump blood to keep you alive during sleep; the diaphragm, to keep you breathing; and the eyes, which sleep researchers observe dart around during REM sleep—researchers aren't sure why.

Our paleolithic ancestors actually only needed six hours of sleep a night.[19] Today, we barely get by on eight. The difference is this: our ancestors slept better and more efficiently than we do today. Their airways didn't collapse so they weren't interrupted by sleep-disordered breathing. The body has a reflex when it feels satisfied from sleep, and our ancestors reached that threshold sooner than we do now.

Signs of Interrupted Sleep Breathing (Muscle Activation):

➡ Twisted bed sheets in the morning
➡ Dry mouth
➡ Morning headaches
➡ Teeth grinding (bruxism)
➡ Tossing and turning
➡ Limb movement while sleeping

In this chapter, I'm going to introduce a new measurement that I think is just as important as your cholesterol and blood pressure to having a clear picture of your health: *sleep ability*. Sleep ability is how well you're able to breathe without interruptions while you sleep at night. Does your airway stay open and allow airflow even when it narrows during deep sleep? Or does it not have enough space to allow for perfect, uninterrupted airflow? These questions can certainly even determine your cholesterol and blood pressure, as well as your overall health and well-being.

---

19   Gandhi Yetish, Hillard Kaplan, Michael Gurven, Brian Wood, Herman Pontzer, Paul R. Manger, Charles Wilson, Ronald McGregor, and Jerome M. Siegel, "Natural Sleep and Its Seasonal Variations in Three Pre-industrial Societies," Current Biology, (2015) doi: *http://dx.doi.org/10.1016/j.cub.2015.09.046*

Sleep ability is different for everyone. It's partially based on your genetics, but it is more affected by what you were exposed to as a child. Anything that negatively impacts the development of the mouth, jaw, or face can impact your sleep ability.

Factors That Affect Your Sleep Ability

As a child:

➡ Orthodontic treatment, if not done with consideration of the airway, can make the airway narrower

➡ Crowded or crooked teeth indicate a narrowing in the mouth and thus a narrowing in the airway

➡ Prolonged bottle-feeding, thumb-sucking, or sippy cups, which don't promote proper growth of the face and jaw because they train unnatural sucking motion

➡ Allergies, which block the nasal passages and force mouth breathing

➡ A diet composed of packaged, easy-to-digest foods

➡ Prolonged thumb sucking

➡ C-section; vaginal births affect facial development, meaning it could be a factor in airway development

As an adult:

➡ A large tongue

➡ Small neck

➡ Receding or "weak" chin

➡ Allergies

➡ Difficulty breathing through the nose

➡ BMI (body mass index)

➡ A large neck circumference

Why Not All Sleep is Created Equal

*The amount of sleep required by the average person
is five more minutes.*
—*Wilson Mizner*

*I never get enough sleep. I stay up late at night because I'm Night
Guy. Night Guy wants to stay up late. What about getting up after
five hours of sleep? Oh, that's Morning Guy's problem. That's not my
problem. I'm Night Guy. I stay up as late as I want. So you get up
in the morning with the alarm, you're exhausted, you're groggy. You
hate that guy! See, Night Guy always screws Morning Guy.*
—*Jerry Seinfeld*

Get your eight hours. This is what we are told by doctors, nutritionists, and government agencies. As long as you're getting your eight hours and sleeping through the night, you're in the clear. Unfortunately, good sleep isn't that simple or guaranteed.

When I ask my patients not just how *many hours* they're sleeping, but how *well* they're sleeping, they assure me, "Oh, I'm sleeping fine!" or "I'm a great sleeper!" and "I try to get eight hours a night." In reality, we are *terrible* judges of our own sleep quality.

I would say roughly 9 out of 10 of my patients who've had a sleep-disordered breathing diagnosis thought they were sleeping fine before their diagnosis. Many of them consider themselves good sleepers since they can sleep anywhere, they can nap, or they sleep a lot. But if there's anything to take away from this book, it's this: you cannot objectively say how well you're sleeping.

Reasons We Are Terrible Judges of Our Own Sleep Quality

1. **We don't know what we're missing.** Our baseline is poor sleep. Because much of our sleep ability is determined by how our faces and airways grow during childhood, we don't know what a good night's sleep actually feels like. When you've never experienced something, you can't know what you're missing.

2. **Changes in our sleep ability are subtle.** Changes in the quality of our sleep are often so subtle and gradual that we can't perceive them. This is something that happened to me. I accepted my tiredness as a normal part of aging and being a busy father of three with a growing practice. I was performing well during my waking hours, so it never once crossed my mind that there could be a problem.

Add a frog to a pot of boiling water, and he will jump out immediately. But if you add a frog to room temperature water that is slowly brought to boil, he will never jump out to save himself. When my patients tell me, "Well, but I have tons of energy" or "I feel fine" or "I don't snore," I am reminded of this old story.

3. **Good health disguises suboptimal sleep.** The body can overcompensate extraordinarily well for poor sleep—which is why energy levels aren't very good at telling us much except when it comes to the later stages of sleep-disordered breathing.

But the physiological changes that occur due to interrupted sleep aren't going to impact your health tomorrow; they take decades to accumulate.

4. We treat sleep like it's automatic. We do a lot of things when it comes to getting healthy, but rarely do we think about our sleep *quality*. Sleep is innate, but it's not guaranteed.

It's hard to know how well we're sleeping, which is a large part of why up to 70 million Americans have an untreated sleep breathing condition. Couple this with the fact that most of us have been exposed to factors in our environment that narrow the airway—things like allergies, orthodontic treatment, pharmaceutical drugs, obesity, and the modern diet—and you get a condition that is extremely common, yet extremely invisible.

Range of Sleep-Disordered Breathing

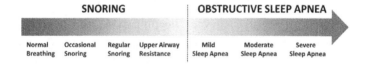

It's not just sleep apnea—sleep apnea is a small part of the wide spectrum of sleep-disordered breathing. All of our work in medicine is on the far right-hand side of this spectrum. When my patients tell me, "Oh, I don't have sleep apnea," I say, "That could be right, but I'm talking about taking care of you now, while your symptoms are still mild. Let's take care of you *before you get sleep apnea.*"

Patients who have seen a sleep doctor come back and tell me, "Oh, I'm within the normal range" or "It's only mild." Mild to moderate sounds benign, doesn't it? The truth is, being anywhere on the spectrum is cause for concern. There are plenty of people who can spend their whole lives in the middle of the spectrum and still suffer, thanks to the cumulative damage of years of sleep-disordered breathing.

Sleep breathing only becomes more difficult with age, and the effects of sleep disruption compound over the decades. Even if you're below the normal range *now*, that could change in a few years—or with a pregnancy or other life event. Sleep breathing is something to manage your whole life—just like cholesterol, blood pressure, and weight.

Instead of "Did I get eight hours?" we should be asking ourselves, "How well did I sleep?" And you can't answer that question without considering your sleep breathing. My patients who insist to me that they're "sleeping fine" and go by these proverbial eight hours are caught in what I call the eight-hour sleep paradox—they're thinking in terms of quantity, not quality. And that's a dangerous place to be.

The Downward Spiral

There's a dangerous, self-perpetuating cycle I see in many of my ambitious, burn-the-candle-at-both-ends patients who are starting families and companies and changing the world. As their sleep breathing gets worse, they have less energy and wherewithal to make sleep a priority again. In many cases, the worse your sleep ability is, the more likely you are to believe that you're fine.

The Cost of Interrupted Sleep Breathing

There's a cost to being awake. Our waking hours are a destructive time, and deep sleep is the only time when your body shuts down one system (your muscles) so it can focus energy on repair. Deep sleep is when the brain promotes cellular regeneration, making your body and mind younger. Deep sleep is when the brain consolidates your memories and the things you learn. It processes emotions. It optimizes important neuronal connections that might otherwise deteriorate due to lack of activity—which is perhaps one of the purposes of dreaming. Deep sleep reorganizes information and works through problems.

Not only is deep sleep essential to functioning at your highest level during your waking hours, but it's also critical for preventing brain problems. Diseases and disorders like Alzheimer's, dementia, depression, anxiety, and schizophrenia are linked to deprivation of deep sleep. The brain uses more energy than any other organ in the body, accounting for 20% of the body's total haul—and when an organ uses a lot of energy, there's a lot of waste produced.

A major function of deep sleep is to clear this waste. In fact, certain neurological conditions such as Alzheimer's are referred to as "dirty brain" diseases because people with these diseases show buildup of a certain waste product (amyloid-beta) in their brains.

Think of it like this: just as we accumulate trash in our homes, every action in our brain and body produces waste. What amyloid-beta buildup means is that the brain is taking out the trash, but no one is coming to pick it up.[20] Sleep is how the brain cleans itself, so when sleep goes awry, so does brain health.

Uninterrupted sleep is also essential to learning and creativity. Researchers have observed that the brain displays the same signature during learning as during deep sleep. Sleep is essential for strengthening memories so that it's easier for you to remember what you learned the day before.[21] If you're a student, those are the items you studied last night that are on tomorrow's exam. It's not uncommon for entrepreneurs, students, scientists, researchers, writers, and other creatives to wake up in the morning realizing that they figured something out in their sleep.

Physiological Activities During Deep Sleep

➡ Cellular regeneration
➡ Cognitive restoration
➡ Memory archival and solidification
➡ Emotional processing
➡ Growth hormone release

---

20   Lulu Xie, Hongyi Kang, Qiwu Xu, Michael J. Chen, Yonghong Liao, Meenakshisunda-ram Thiyagarajan, John O'Donnell, Daniel J. Christensen, Charles Nicholson, Jeffrey J. Iliff, Takahiro Takano, Rashid Deane, and Maiken Nedergaard, "Science Drives Metabolite Clearance from the Adult Brain," *Science* 342, no. 6156 (2013): 373-377, doi:10.1126/science.1241224.

21   Arwen Curry, "Catching Up on Sleep Science." *QUEST Northern California,* 2014, *http:// science.kqed.org/quest/video/catching-up-on-sleep-science/.*

Sleep enhances our...

✓ Athletic performance, making us more energetic, quicker on our feet, and more accurate in our judgments.

✓ Cognitive performance, judgment, memory, creativity, problem-solving skills, ability to deal with stress, ability to interpret social cues, and just about every other cognitive process.

✓ Neurological performance, endocrine balance, and musculoskeletal growth and repair.

✓ Immune system. Good sleep cuts the risk of the common cold.[22] As it turns out, the immune system is most active during deep sleep.

✓ Ability to keep weight off with greater ease and to maintain a healthy weight.

During sleep, blood pressure dips as an opportunity for the cardiovascular system to recover from the demands of the day, so it's no surprise that studies have linked sleep-disordered breathing with heart failure, strokes, and coronary heart disease.[23] If your blood pressure is higher than this dip, even while you're asleep, that's going to add to your long-term risk for heart disease.

---

22   Aric A. Prather, Denise Janicki-Deverts, Martica H. Hall, and Sheldon Cohen, "Behaviorally Assessed Sleep and Susceptibility to the Common Cold," *Sleep* 38, no. 9, *http://dx.doi.org/10.5665/sleep.4968.*

23   Eyal Shahar, Coralyn W. Whitney, Susan Redline, Elisa T. Lee, Anne B. Newman, F. Javier Nieto, George T. O'Connor, Lori L. Boland, Joseph E. Schwartz, and Jonathan M. Samet, "Sleep-disordered Breathing and Cardiovascular Disease," American Journal of Respiratory and Critical Care Medicine 163, no. 1 (2001): 19-25, doi: 10.1164/ajrccm.163.1.2001008.

When it comes to heart health and sleep breathing, I always think of my patients who are athletes. They are young, fit, healthy, and have no signs of any heart trouble whatsoever. They appear to outrun their sleep breathing problems thanks to the great shape they're in, but that's a temporary solution. A small airway always catches up with you.

There has been surprisingly little research when it comes to sleep-disordered breathing and cancer. However, one study, which followed 1,500 participants in Wisconsin, found that interrupted breathing during sleep promoted the growth of cancer tumors and therefore increased risk of death from cancer.[24] Similarly, a study published last year in the *American Journal of Respiratory and Critical Care Medicine* links snoring and sleep-disordered breathing with an increased risk of cancer.[25] The study tracked 1,500 people for 22 years and found that mild or moderate snoring increases your risk of cancer death.[26]

---

24   F. Javier Nieto, Paul E. Peppard, Terry Young, Laurel Finn, Khin Mae Hla, and Ramon Farré, "Sleep-disordered Breathing and Cancer Mortality," *American Journal of Respiratory and Critical Care Medicine* 186, no. 2 (2012): 190-194, doi: 10.1164/rccm.201201-0130OC.

25   Reena Mehra, Emelia J. Benjamin, Eyal Shahar, Daniel J. Gottlieb, Rawan Nawabit. H. Lester Kirchner, Jayakumar Sahadevan, and Susan Redline, "Association of Nocturnal Arrhythmias with Sleep-disordered Breathing: The Sleep Heart Health Study," *American Journal of Respiratory and Critical Care Medicine* 173, no. 8 (2006): 910-916, doi: 10.1164/rccm.200509-1442OC.

26   Cindy Kuzma, "Snoring Linked to Cancer," *Men's Health*, May 25, 2012, http://www.menshealth.com/health/snoring-linked-cancer?category=supplements

When you miss out on deep sleep. . .

✓ Insulin levels rise, and your body stores more fat.

✓ Levels of the hormone that makes you feel full and controls your appetite (leptin) crash, and your body can't melt fat as well.

✓ Appetite-regulating hormones go haywire, making us hungrier and making us crave unhealthy foods.

✓ Testosterone levels sink, as do your libido and muscle-building ability.

✓ HGH (human growth hormone) levels shrink, taking away your body's natural anti-aging ability. As obsessed as we are with looking young, we are missing out on the best anti-aging treatment there is. As far as age-defying serums go, sleep is the best stuff out there, thanks to HGH, which is produced in stage 3 delta wave deep sleep and is essential for healing damaged tissues.

When you get your needed deep sleep . . .

✓ The body scavenges for harmful chemicals in your body and removes them.

✓ Aging cells are repaired.

✓ Muscles and other tissues are repaired.

✓ Insulin levels are regulated[27] and glucose and testosterone levels are stabilized.

---

27   E. Tasali, R. Leproult, D.A. Ehrmann, and E. Van Cauter, "Slow-wave sleep and the risk of type 2 diabetes in humans," *Proceedings of the National Academy of Sciences of the United States of America* 105, no. 3 (2008): 1044-1049, doi: 10.1073/pnas.0706446105.

✓ The immune system is restored.

✓ Hormones ghrelin and leptin, which play a role in appetite, are stabilized.

In children, HGH is responsible for helping the body grow and develop. In adults, it's essential to all of the above activities as well as for keeping you young, which it does by allowing the body to renew and restore itself. Every day, our bodies are aging and dying. HGH is the only thing we have on our side to slow this process down. HGH is released only during deep sleep, and interruptions to deep sleep stop its release. It's no surprise that some people call HGH the fountain of youth!

It's hard not to find a system that isn't affected by sleep deprivation. After two months of treating his small airway and sleeping better than ever, one of my patients came in for a checkup. He described poor sleep this way: "You become pissed off, overweight, hungry, and depressed." That just about sums it up.

Symptoms of Interrupted Sleep Breathing

➡ Aches and spasms, especially in the head or neck
➡ Aging too rapidly
➡ Allergies
➡ Anxiety
➡ Arthritis
➡ Bedwetting
➡ Brain fog

➡ Broken teeth, TMD (temporomandibular joint dysfunction), jaw pain, lock jaw

➡ Craving junky carbohydrates and looking to food and coffee for energy

➡ Decision-making difficulty

➡ Decreased motivation and drive

➡ Depressed mood

➡ Dry skin

➡ Eczema

➡ Fatigue

➡ Feeling overwhelmed

➡ Focusing difficulty

➡ Heart problems

➡ Insulin resistance

➡ Irritability

➡ Joint pain

➡ Lightheadedness

➡ Low energy

➡ Memory issues

➡ Nausea

➡ Needing to get up in the middle of the night to urinate

➡ Negative thoughts

➡ Not thriving

➡ Reaction time increased

➡ Sexual dysfunction, erectile dysfunction (ED), or lowered sex drive

➡ Sleepiness after meals

➡ Sleepiness in the afternoon

➡ Thyroid issues

You don't have to be sleepy to be affected! In fact, a lot of healthy people easily overcompensate for sleep deprivation. It might feel like you have energy, but your body can't keep it up forever. You can't be on top of your game without deep sleep. If you're a child, you won't reach your academic and behavioral potential. If you're a doctor, you'll be scraping by, and work will be a lot harder than it needs to be. If you're a businessperson, it'll take all your energy to get through the day, and you won't have energy left when you get home. If you're an athlete and your body isn't repairing itself at night, your heart and muscles aren't getting a chance to rest and repair, and you won't be able to build as much muscle and endurance.

How a Small Airway Makes You Grind Your Teeth

If you ask ten different dentists, "What causes grinding?" prepare yourself for several different answers: stress, how the teeth come together, hormonal fluctuations, and so on. These answers aren't wrong; grinding is multifactorial—meaning it's caused by a perfect storm of factors working together.

There is one thing, however, that we are beginning to understand: there is a connection between grinding and sleep breathing. The latest studies suggest that grinding is an instinctual response by your body when you have trouble breathing. Grinding pushes your jaw forward to get your tongue out of the way to open up your airway, which helps you breathe.[28]

---

28   G.D. Klasser, N. Rei, and G.J. Lavigne, "Sleep bruxism etiology: the evolution of a changing paradigm," *Canadian Dental Association* 81, no. 2 (2015), http://europepmc.org/abstract/med/25633110

This might explain why we see fetuses grind in the womb. Fetuses don't have teeth and aren't breathing air, yet they display a back-and-forth motion with their jaws when oxygen levels to the brain drop. Could this be an instinctual motion we have evolved as a species to prevent us from choking to death while we sleep?

Whether or not this is the case, if you're grinding your teeth, your muscles are online and active, meaning you are not in deep-stage sleep. Each time you grind, your brain bounces into a lighter stage of sleep. Everyone thinks of the lungs when it comes to breathing, but in this case, the masseter (your chewing muscle) is an important muscle of respiration.

All of the signs and symptoms of a sleep breathing disorder were present in my father. He was hyperactive—counterintuitively, a sign of a sleep breathing disorder; his body was overcompensating for lack of deep sleep. He was a severe teeth grinder, perhaps because of stress, but also as a response to trying to reopen his airway. He had a small, narrow roof of the mouth and crowded teeth—a sign of a narrow airway due to a small apartment and normal-sized furniture, to use our analogy. He needed naps. Despite having a strong jaw, he was retrognathic—that is, he had what you might call an "overbite," a jaw that was further back in position and a chin that sloped down into the neck without a lot of definition in the profile.

I am convinced that my father's brain and spinal column weren't getting a chance to repair thanks to interrupted sleep breathing. The fact that he slept eight hours each night simply wasn't enough.

Sleep Is Not a Sign of Weakness

Being a dentist is sometimes like being a hairdresser. My patients see me more frequently than their general practitioner, and we always have in-depth conversations about how things are really going—the brain fog, the unexplained weight gain, the trouble focusing or remembering names and facts, the morning headaches. My private practice is in the Silicon Valley, so my patients are some of the most stressed-out, burned-out, and sleep-deprived people out there. The thing I always must explain to my patients is that being sleep deprived is not a sign of weakness or something you need to push through. Our culture praises people who don't give up in the face of struggle and hardship, but sometimes we take our "no pain, no gain" culture a little too far—especially when it comes to sleep. I have patients who are shocked to discover that they don't have to have a short temper, difficulty maintaining their weight, or trouble focusing; they just had trouble sleep breathing. "I didn't realize that my life didn't have to be so hard," one patient told me after just three weeks of treatment.

What Deep Sleep Looks Like

There's a mobile app that I ask my patients to download when I suspect sleep breathing issues. The app was recommended to me by a sleep medicine neurologist. Before you get into bed, you turn the app on, and it listens throughout the night for any noise. If there's a noise, it records it. If there's silence, the app doesn't record. Upon waking up, the app tells you the number of interruptions during the night and a playback of every sound the app picked up.[29]

---

29   The app's called Sleep Analyzer, and you can find it here: *https://itunes.apple.com/us/app/sleep-analyzer/id296266786?mt=8*. There are other, similar apps out there if that one doesn't work with your phone. For more information, you can learn more on my website, *askthedentist.com.* "How to Find Out If You're Sleeping Well," *http://askthedentist.com/how-to-find-out-sleeping-well/.* I discuss apps more later.

My patients often come back to me shocked at the number of interruptions they got, which can go into the hundreds. One of my patients heard herself moan every time the dog shook its collar. Another heard that the air conditioning came on in the middle of the night and made an awful noise. People hear themselves coughing, snorting, gasping, grinding, tossing, and turning; and most times, these noises come as a complete shock. How could they be making those noises when they felt like they slept through the entire night peacefully?

Sometimes, I'll have patients tell me, "Dr. B, a small airway isn't the problem. The problem is I always have to go to the bathroom in the middle of the night. *That's* what's interrupting my sleep." Waking up in the middle of the night to go to the bathroom is incredibly frustrating and fragments sleep, but the cause isn't what most people think. Needing to go to the bathroom in the middle of the night is actually a sign that you're not in deep sleep. In deep sleep, a hormone called ADH is secreted to prevent you from needing to urinate. As you can imagine, if you're not able to stay in deep sleep, ADH can't be secreted normally, so you'll be woken up needing to urinate.

During a night of true, uninterrupted deep sleep, you won't have to wake up in the middle of the night to go to the bathroom because ADH is on board.[30] When you're in deep sleep, you don't hear your partner flushing the toilet or the dog barking outside. You're not too hot or too cold—you're completely knocked out.

---

30   Helene Kemmer, Alexander M. Mathes, Olaf Dilk, Andreas Gröschel, Christian Grass, and Micheal Stöckle, "Obstructive Sleep Apnea Syndrome Is Associated with Overactive Bladder and Urgency Incontinence in Men," Sleep 32, no. 2 (2009): 271-275, http://www.ncbi.nlm.nih.gov/pmc/articles/PMC2635592/

Deep sleep is still and silent. When you wake up, you have no memory of the night before, and it feels as if no time has passed.

The Emotional Impact of Fighting for Your Life

Breathing interruptions during sleep also take an emotional toll. Imagine this: your brain is in deep sleep, beginning its repair cycle, when suddenly it senses a breathing difficulty. The brain is startled out of deep sleep into lighter sleep to roll you over, turn your neck, grind your teeth, or open your mouth in order to start breathing again.

This panic mode saves your life, but not without a cost to your emotional health. We wake up with a subconscious memory of this awful stress. It makes us anxious, remembering the feelings but not what happened.

Over time, all this stress on the body makes us sick. You might say that we do pretty well considering, but at some point, the question becomes, how much panic and stress can you take?

The fight-or-flight response puts wear and tear on the body. When chronically activated, the adrenal gland, which produces the panic hormone, becomes weak and leads to you feeling rundown, overwhelmed, and generally unwell. When this happens, other hormones try to compensate, and the whole system goes awry—setting the stage for adrenal fatigue, chronic fatigue, and thyroid trouble.

I have many patients with depression, anxiety, and other psychological conditions who find that treatment of their sleep breathing allows them to be far less reliant on drugs.

After treating my own sleep breathing, I found that I had much more patience with my daughters. I used to feel like my temper was too short with them and that after work, I just didn't have the energy to handle things. Now I realize that being emotionally panicked multiple times each night was impacting my capacity for patience and empathy in my waking hours. Having more patience is one of the best side effects of sleep breathing treatment that I've experienced.

I used to think that modern medicine would one day cure neurological diseases with a new drug. But the cure we need is an old one: sleep.

Quality sleep is what allows us to be the kind, emotionally available, and loving human beings we all want to be. It puts us in control of our lives and our destinies.

Chapter 3:
A New Approach to Reverse
This Epidemic

Each patient carries his or her own doctor inside him or her.
—Albert Schweitzer

We can't solve problems by using the same kind of thinking we used
when we created them.
—Albert Einstein

An ounce of prevention is worth a pound of cure.
—Unknown

Ideally, we'd end the book right here. By now, you know about the importance of sleep breathing as well as your risk factors for sleep-disordered breathing and what this means for your health. But how does one actually start breathing better?

Unfortunately, our healthcare system isn't set up in a way that makes this easy.

At first, this dumbfounded me. I would refer a patient who showed signs of sleep-disordered breathing to a sleep specialist, and off they'd go. But when I'd see them six months later in the dental chair and ask them how it went with the sleep study, over and over again, I would get the same reply:

"Oh, they told me I look too healthy for a sleep study."

"My doctor said grinding my teeth isn't enough to qualify for a sleep study."

That's when I started to dig in to help my patients push through the barriers in the medical system to get sleep studies, get treatment, and get that treatment covered by insurance. I began to learn a lot about the rules of the game.

This book is not just about awareness for sleep-disordered breathing; it's also a guide for doing something about it. That's exactly what the three-step approach is all about.

Understanding the Three Steps to Treating Sleep Ability

The three steps are:

1. Measure: Just as you and your doctor monitor your cholesterol and blood pressure, I will show you how to measure your sleep ability.

2. Treat: There are simple, comfortable, and convenient ways to keep your airway open at night. I'll show you how to know which way is right for you.

3. Verify: Very often, people who experience treatment are amazed at what they were missing. This step is essential to quantify how much your treatment is helping your sleep and, since sleep ability gets worse with age, how to tweak your treatment as time goes by.

We'll discuss these in detail over the next three chapters and then dive into the insurance issue.

Chapter 4:
Step 1: Measure

When I woke up this morning, my girlfriend asked me, 'Did you sleep good?' I said, 'No, I made a few mistakes.'
—Steven Wright

Laura knew something didn't feel quite right. She felt foggy, tired, anxious, and depressed. Her doctor believed Laura's symptoms were caused by depression, so Laura was prescribed drugs. Unbeknownst to Laura and her doctor, her real problem was that she wasn't breathing properly at night.

Laura began to feel better with her medication, but every night while she slept, her adrenal glands were being worn down by sleep interruptions, and every morning, she woke up anxious and tired. Since her adrenal glands were in overdrive at night, they couldn't function properly during the day, and she couldn't handle all the little crises that cropped up—like running late or a boss putting pressure on her. As the years went by and the gradual damage on her body worsened, Laura needed to increase the dosage of her medication.

Finally, when Laura moved to California and came into my office for the first time at age 43, I could see the red flags for sleep-disordered breathing. She had wear and tear on her teeth that told me she was grinding. I could hear Laura's breathing becoming labored as she lay flat on her back in the dental chair.

People like Laura often end up bounced around from specialist to specialist, who are trained to offer medication or surgery to solve diseases in general; but the underlying cause is sleep-disordered breathing, which undercuts the body's ability to do its essential repair work each night. Treating the symptoms may relieve things short-term, but long-term, the symptoms keep coming back.

I explained to Laura that I saw in her some of the early red flags for a sleep breathing disorder and recommended she see her doctor for a sleep study referral. Even though Laura didn't fit the typical profile for sleep apnea, I was able to see the early signs while she sat in the dental chair.

More and more, dentists are the ones screening for sleep-disordered breathing. The earliest signs of sleep breathing issues appear in the mouth. Your dentist sees you more often than your doctor (every six months), and is more likely to see you in a reclined position than sitting upright.

How the face and jaw develop during childhood impacts the size of the airway, so it's up to dentists to teach patients about a small airway and consider the size of the airway when making recommendations or doing orthodontic treatment.

Public knowledge and education are still catching up to the science. Sleep breathing is not a topic usually covered in dental school and medical schools still teach doctors to look only for the end-stage signs of sleep apnea, such as obesity and falling asleep at the wheel. Screening for the early signs of sleep breathing problems at both the dentist and doctor isn't yet commonplace, but it will be one day with efforts of organizations like the AADSM (American Academy of Dental Sleep Medicine) and AASM (American Academy of Sleep Medicine).

Here's what to ask your dentist at your next check-up:

What to Ask for at a Dental Screening:

1. Ask if you grind your teeth. If you're grinding at night, whatever the reason, it means your muscles are active and you're not in deep sleep.

2. Ask if you have lingual erosion of the upper (maxillary) teeth. If so, that means acid is getting pushed up by the tongue at night because you're lying backwards.

3. Ask if you have a scalloped tongue. This is something you might be able to identify yourself by looking at your tongue in the mirror—does your tongue have any teeth marks on the sides? This happens when the adjacent teeth compress the tongue, leaving their mark. A scalloped tongue is a red flag for sleep-disordered breathing. 70% of people with a scalloped tongue have obstructive sleep apnea. Also ask if you have a fissured tongue, which has a groove down the middle of the tongue, indicating that the tongue doesn't have enough room in the mouth and is folding over on itself.

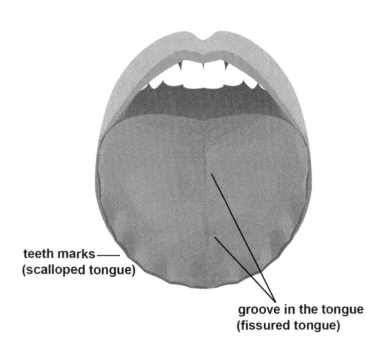

teeth marks——
(scalloped tongue)

groove in the tongue
(fissured tongue)

4. Ask for a Mallampati or Friedman Score. All you have to do is stick your tongue out while your dentist examines the anatomy of the back of your throat. If he or she can see your tonsils and the beginning of your airway, you're less likely to have sleep-disordered breathing than if all your dentist can see is your tongue (see figure below). The Friedman's classification is similar to the Mallampati, except the assessment is done with the tongue in a position closer to its natural position during sleep.[31]

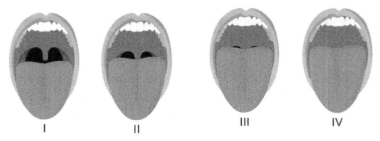

Mallampati Classifications: Type I is less likely to have sleep-disordered breathing than Types II, III, and IV.

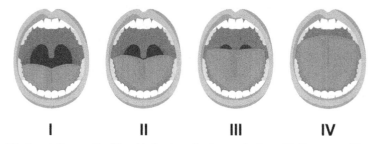

Friedman's Tongue Position: Notice how the tongue is viewed in its rest position.

---

31   M. Friedman, C. Hamilton, C.G. Samuelson, M.E. Lundgren, T. Pott, "Diagnostic value of the Friedman tongue position and Mallampati classification for obstructive sleep apnea: a meta-analysis," Otolaryngol Head Neck Surg 148, no. 4 (2013): 540-547, doi: 10.1177/0194599812473413

5. Ask your dentist if you have a large tongue. The larger your tongue is, the more it pushes down on the hyoid bone, which narrows the airway.

Some dentists will take a three-dimensional x-ray of your airway to assess your risk of sleep-disordered breathing. The jury is still out on the accuracy of these x-rays in predicting your risk, as there isn't enough evidence to support them.[32] They record the airway in its awake state and remember, the muscles behave differently while awake and while asleep.

Starting Off Small: Measuring Sleep at Home

If a sleep study feels overwhelming, you're not quite ready for it yet, or it's prohibitively expensive, there are some ways you can get started.

The first thing I recommend is downloading a mobile app that records the sounds you make while you sleep. It will record noises above a certain threshold of ambient noise and only play back to you sounds that went above that threshold.

Some people are surprised to play it back in the morning to hear they had 10, 15, even 80 interruptions. They hear all sorts of things—like snoring, sleep talking, kicking, tossing and turning, and moaning. All of these sounds are indications that deep sleep may have been interrupted because, remember, if muscles are activated, your body can't be in deep sleep.

Using an app to start with is an easy first step to get a baseline; you can even start tonight. Depending on what you hear during

---

32   N.A. Alsufyani, C. Flores-Mir, and P.W. Major, "Three-dimensional segmentation of the upper airway using cone beam CT: a systematic review," Dentomaxillofac Radiology 41, no. 4 (2012): 276–284, doi: 10.1259/dmfr/79433138

the night, you can make a guess about your sleep ability—although, keep in mind, this is not a replacement for a sleep study or seeing your doctor. But if you've ever wondered what's going on at night, an app that records the noises you make can be a good start to get clues. You can also use results from an app like this to bring to your doctor to make the case for a proper sleep study.

Fitness Trackers and Apps: How Accurate Are They?

As a tech geek myself, I hate to say it, but the verdict is in: sleep experts across the board agree that these apps are not sophisticated enough to report any meaningful insights about sleep. There are a lot of sleep apps out there that claim to measure sleep, but the only apps that are worth using for now are the ones that record the sounds you make.

Apps that claim to measure your sleep stages are the most misleading, since this is impossible—sleep stages are determined by brain waves, which a mobile phone can't measure. These apps are masquerading as sleep studies, and the sleep reports and graphs they generate are inaccurate. The same goes for accelerometers and watches like Fitbit and Apple Watch.

Instead, use an app that records the sounds you make while you sleep and plays only those sounds back to you in the morning—this does not replace a sleep study or a diagnosis by a sleep physician, but it is a good way to get started in understanding what's going on at night. Examples include Sleep Talk Recorder for Android and Sleep Analyzer for iOS.

I have no doubt that smartphone apps will be at the center of the digital revolution for healthcare, but as of right now, the technology isn't there. One of my patients, Tricia, loves checking her Fitbit because it reminds her that her MAD (mandibular advancement device— a retainer-like device that can help keep the airway open during sleep discussed in Chapter 5) is working. In this way, apps and other trackers can be great for motivation, but they can't be used to rule out sleep-disordered breathing.

Other Things to Check At Home:

1. Take a mirror and a flashlight (or use bright daylight) to look inside your mouth. If you haven't had them removed, your tonsils should be visible. If you see the tonsils fall into your airway space, there is less room to breathe—another red flag for sleep-disordered breathing.

2. See if you can breathe through your nose. It's something we often don't think about, but the mouth was never designed to do the breathing, the nose is. When you're not breathing through you nose, your blood is not getting all the oxygen it needs to function properly. Check in with yourself throughout the day—while on your computer, while sitting watching TV, while driving—is your mouth open or closed? If it's open, you're not breathing through your nose.

Mouth Taping and the Buteyko Breathing Method

Add this to the list of things that sound weird but really work: Mouth taping is the practice of sleeping with the lips taped closed. If you're thinking, "but how will I breathe?" know this: nasal breathing is the correct and optimal way to breathe. It makes the lungs more efficient at breathing, helps avoid heartburn and GERD, and even puts the brain into a state of relaxation. Nose breathing increases the production of nitric oxide, which lowers heart rate, increases circulation, and is integral in protecting organs from damage. Close to 80% of the Western population is breathing incorrectly through the mouth, elevating blood pressure and heart rate, worsening asthma, allergies, and depriving the heart, brain, and other organs of optimal oxygenation. The nose—not the mouth—is designed for breathing. There is no reason why you shouldn't

---

be able to breathe through your nose while completely at rest in bed. If you wake up in the morning with the tape still covering your lips, you are a capable nose breather! If not, then you know you need to see your ENT because there's an obstruction in your nose.

A lot of people sleep like this every night to promote proper breathing habits, and even say they feel better in the morning when they tape. How to do it: lightly tape your lips closed while in the rest position and go to sleep. Use a surgical tape like SnorLess Strips so you don't have any marks on your face in the morning. Fold one side of the tape so you have a pull-off tab.

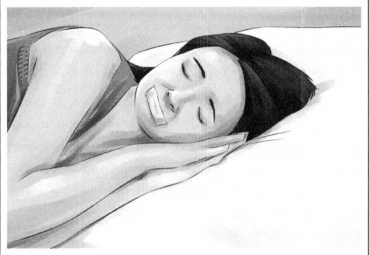

Mouth taping is the practice of sleeping with the lips taped closed to promote nose breathing, which has many health benefits.

Working With Your Doctor

Looking for signs at home and seeing your dentist are a good start, but never replace seeing a sleep specialist and getting a diagnosis. Sleep-disordered breathing and sleep apnea are diagnosed only by physicians who specialize in sleep medicine. In most cases, you will have to see your general practitioner physician to get a referral to a sleep specialist.

The Epworth Sleepiness Scale (ESS) is, at the moment, the way that medicine decides whether you get to have a sleep study. Unfortunately, much of what the ESS measures is relevant for later-stage symptoms—making it less useful for catching early warning signs. "The ESS was never designed as a sole instrument to determine whether a patient is or is not sleepy for the purpose of approving diagnostic testing"[33] and has been criticized by sleep specialists. Studies have shown that many patients who had sleep apnea didn't fall asleep in the situations listed in the ESS.[34]

While the ESS isn't sensitive enough to be an effective diagnostic tool,[35] I've included it in Appendix C since it's likely the first thing you'll come across when talking to your doctor about your sleep. Consider it a starting point, and don't be afraid to push your doctor for a sleep study or to confront him or her if you don't agree with his or her decision.

---

33   Stuart F. Quan, "Abuse of the Epworth Sleepiness Scale," Journal of Clinical Sleep Medicine 9, no. 10 (2013): 987, doi: 10.5664/jcsm.3062.

34   Anh Tu Duy Nguyen, Marc A. Baltzan, David Small, Norman Wolkove, Simone Guillon, Mark Palayew, "Clinical Reproducibility of the Epworth Sleepiness Scale," *Journal of Clinical Sleep Medicine* 2, no. 2 (2006): 170-174, *http://www.aasmnet.org/jcsm/Articles/020210.pdf*.

35   Damien Leger, "A Socioeconomic Perspective of Sleep Disorders (Insomnia and Obstructive Sleep Apnea)," *The Oxford Handbook of Sleep and Sleep Disorders*, ed. Charles M. Morin and Colin A. Espie (Oxford University Press, 2012), 334.

A Note on Choosing the Right Doctor for You

I've had many patients tell me they brought their symptoms to their doctor, who did not believe them or just wanted to prescribe a pill instead of getting to the root of the issue. One woman, Eleanor, had her family doctor prescribe her statins when she started to have high blood pressure at age 23. There are plenty of situations where statins are appropriate, but starting on statins at such a young age would have set up Eleanor for a lifetime of side effects from the drug.

Many doctors are trained to see symptoms and prescribe a pharmaceutical drug for those symptoms. The problem with this approach is that it deals with the symptom but not the root cause of that symptom. You can keep replacing flat tires, but what if the real problem is a nail in the driveway? Make sure that every healthcare practitioner you see is concerned with treating not just your symptoms but also the root cause of those symptoms. This is called functional or integrative medicine.

Furthermore, most doctors are so squeezed that they can spend only fifteen minutes with you. Discussing sleep breathing takes longer than that.

What you can do to help this is to give your doctor more data points than just the ESS. Besides how you respond on the ESS, bring the checklist of information included in Appendix E to your appointment with your sleep specialist. This checklist is a list of factors that should be considered by your doctor in determining whether or not you get a sleep study. The ESS isn't good enough by itself.

Side note: another common ESS alternative is the STOP BANG questionnaire, included in Appendix E. Several studies show that the STOP BANG is more effective than the ESS because it is more sensitive and more readily able to pick out sleep-disordered breathing. Take both and compare them, and give this information to your doctor.

Getting Blocked from a PSG Prescription

One of my patients, Adam, came into an appointment extremely upset. His doctor wouldn't prescribe him a sleep study. The doctor's rationale: Adam was young (age 26), healthy, had a low BMI, and had only one symptom. The symptom? Adam was a severe grinder. He would wake up in the middle of the night, and he suffered from anxiety and headaches. We worked together with his primary care physician to convince her that Adam needed a sleep test. Sleep tests are expensive, so there are systems in place to limit the number prescribed.

Insurance companies and hospitals have business units that are constantly analyzing how many people get these studies and how to keep costs low. Some large medical health organizations, HMOs, and PPOs have incentives for doctors not to prescribe too many expensive tests, including sleep studies and MRIs. These incentives include allowing doctors to split the money saved and even go so far as to publish a list of which doctors prescribe the most sleep tests each month. It's logical for doctors to pick the healthiest-looking and youngest patient as the one to deny a test. This protects them from liability.

The key is to know how the system works, know the rules, and how to get yourself the care you need and deserve within that system.

The PSG: The Gold Standard[36]

If you score a 9 or higher on the ESS or demonstrate your need for a sleep study using the checklist in Appendix E, your doctor will start you off with a prescription for a sleep study to try to understand what's going on while you sleep.

Ah, but what kind of sleep study? There are several different types of sleep tests, and more are coming out all the time.

The difference is in what data points they record. The most advanced sleep tests are best because they measure pretty much everything—your heart rate, brain waves, nasal pressure, snoring, breathing movements, leg movements, body position, teeth grinding and jaw clenching, oxygen levels, and more. The least advanced tests are cheaper, but they measure only one or two things, don't provide enough data to diagnose sleep conditions, and often lead to inaccurate diagnoses since they under report on the severity of sleep-disordered breathing

Here's really all you need to know:

The only sleep study that is worthwhile and accurate is the polysomnography (PSG). You should do everything you can to get this type of test. When it comes to an accurate diagnosis, a sleep specialist really needs all the data points in a PSG. The simpler tests just don't cut it.

---

36   Throughout, I use "sleep study" and "sleep test" interchangeably. These refer to the same thing, which is some sort of test, PSG or not, that measures two or more data points during sleep.

If You Can't Afford a Sleep Study

If you don't have insurance, you can look into becoming a participant in a research study. Many medical schools are looking for people willing to join a clinical trial as part of their sleep research. ClinicalTrials.gov is a website maintained by the U.S. National Institutes of Health and lets you search for terms like "sleep study" or "polysomnography" plus the area where you live. This is a great way to get a proper sleep study for free or maybe even get paid for it.

The Pitfalls of Non-PSG Sleep Tests

Any test that doesn't measure brain wave patterns can't report on sleep stages. This is important because a sleep specialist needs to be able to see breathing events in relationship to the stage of sleep you're in. Without seeing sleep stages, the tests frequently result in false negatives—indicating there isn't sleep-disordered breathing or that it's milder than it actually is.

These are the two main ways non-PSG studies underreport:

1. One parameter that many of these tests rely on is the oxygen saturation of your blood throughout the night. This is problematic because *you do not need to have low O_2 levels to have sleep-disordered breathing.* Unattended sleep studies can lead to false negatives, and many experts consider them as inferior or bogus. But, alas, they're cheaper and therefore more commonly prescribed.

2. Another way these simplistic tests underestimate sleep breathing issues is by reporting an average AHI (Apnea—Hypopnea Index). Your AHI is the number of times your breathing

either stopped or had some resistance averaged out per hour over the entire night's sleep. An AHI of 1 means you stopped breathing once every hour. However, AHIs are usually highest during REM sleep. People with mild sleep disordered breathing often have an AHI of 0 for all stages of sleep except for REM, when their AHI jumps to 10 or even higher. The average AHI that a simplistic test spits out is under 5, considered "normal." Here's the problem, though: a high AHI during REM means you're being interrupted in the most healing, restorative stage of sleep. Artificially low scores like this give us a false sense of security. Simplistic tests can't measure sleep stages, so they report an average AHI for the whole night—often giving an artificially low score.[37]

Do everything you can to push for a proper PSG; otherwise, you'll never know if you're actually fine or if your sleep-disordered breathing wasn't picked up by the more rudimentary test.

The Night of the PSG: What to Expect

For some people, having to sleep while hooked up to wires and while being watched is an unpleasant idea, but I'd encourage you to look at it this way: it's only one night, and the person watching you isn't a creep! He or she is a trained specialist reporting on your sleep breathing. It's an incredible thing to have so much great data about your sleep!

---

37   If you want to know more about the standards for in-home tests, you can read this study: Nancy A. Collop, W. McDowell Anderson, Brian Boehlecke, David Claman, Rochelle Goldberg, Daniel J. Gottlieb, David Hudgel, Michael Sateia, and Richard Schwab, "Clinical Guidelines for the Use of Unattended Portable Monitors in the Diagnosis of Obstructive Sleep Apnea in Adult Patients: Portable Monitoring Task Force of the American Academy of Sleep Medicine," *Journal of Clinical Sleep Medicine* 3, no. 7 (2007): 737-747; 1-5, *http://www.aasmnet.org/resources/clinicalguidelines/030713.pdf.*

Not only that, but PSGs aren't what most people think. You're not in a glass laboratory being watched by people in lab coats. PSGs are often conducted in sleep centers, where you'll get your own hotel room, complete with a bathroom and cable TV. Some PSGs can even be done in your own home. A sleep technician will come to your home the evening before and morning after to set you up with the test and then remove it and return it to the sleep lab.

The evening before, a technician will hook you up with wires. All the wires connected to your body can be uncomfortable, especially if you're a light sleeper. But don't be put off by this! It may be inconvenient, *but none of those things will alter your sleep test results.*

When you wake up in the morning, the technician will knock on the door, come in, and remove all the wires. Voila, you're done! The data will be sent to your sleep specialist physician for interpretation and diagnosis.

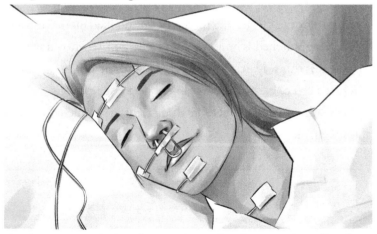

A polysomnography is a sleep study used to diagnose sleep disorders. It may also be used to help adjust and optimize your treatment plan.

The most common question I'm asked about the PSG is: *Is it worth it?* If there is any doubt that your sleep is being interrupted, yes, it's absolutely imperative that you do it. If you have medical insurance and are able to afford this study, then it's easier to stomach. Check with your insurance company to see what kind of coverage it offers. You might be surprised at how affordable a sleep test actually is. If you don't have coverage, work with your doctor to find options. You're not alone. Often, clinics offer highly reduced prices for people who don't have insurance. Similarly, you could get a PSG by being a participant in a clinical study—in which case, the PSG could be something that you get *paid* to do!

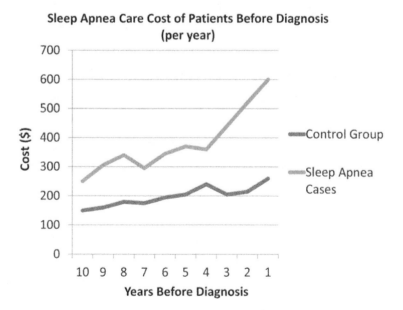

Sleep Apnea Care Cost of Patients Before Diagnosis (per year)

Trying to Pass the Test

When I first signed up to take a sleep study, long before I became a dental sleep medicine dentist, I was in denial about the test.

The achiever in me wanted to do well on this test. I felt like I was preparing for an exam for school. I remember scheduling the sleep study with the office manager, trying to choose a day when I would feel "ready." I made sure to schedule the test on a day when I thought I would sleep best. I waited to schedule my sleep study until I felt I could get my circadian rhythm in order.

Don't wait for some optimal moment to take the test. It's pointless because nothing you do to prepare for the sleep study will matter in terms of the data collected.

That's because sleep studies record what your airway does during deep sleep—so whether you have a good night of sleep or not doesn't matter in terms of the data collected. Knowing exactly what happens to your airway and your body during deep-stage sleep, whether it's good news or bad news, is success.

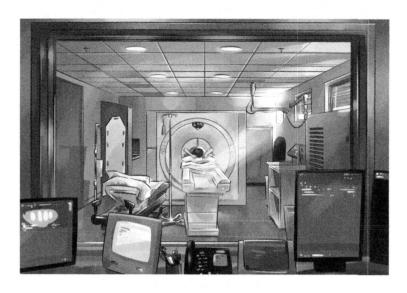

Expectation vs. Reality

The testing bedroom is just like a hotel bedroom with cable TV, Wi-Fi, and a private bathroom. There's an intercom where you can ask for anything you need while you're hooked up—like a glass of water or another blanket.

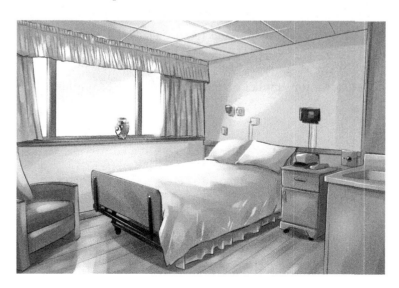

Understanding Your Results

Your next appointment with the sleep medicine specialist will be to go over the data from the study. You will discuss your results and get a diagnosis. Understanding your results is important, so come prepared!

Here's what to know before you go:

✓ Typically, one hour is allotted for this visit. Use all of this time to get your questions answered.

✓ Before your appointment, review and take with you Appendix D, which is a checklist of things to discuss with your doctor and understand about your PSG results.

✓ Get a copy, get a copy, get a copy. I made this mistake the first time I got a PSG. Years later, after joining the AADSM and becoming a sleep dentist and reading my patients' studies, I wanted to reread my own study. It took several phone calls and months to get it mailed to me.

Your sleep specialist considers many factors, but if it were boiled down for simplicity, your diagnosis is based on this:

Apnea-Hypopnea Index (AHI)

AHI	Severity of Sleep-Disordered Breathing
0	Healthy*
0-5	Normal*
5-15	Mild**
15-30	Moderate**
31+	Severe

*Breathing interruptions under 10 seconds are not calculated in AHI. This is why an AHI of zero doesn't rule out Upper Airway Resistance Syndrome (UARS).

**Mild and moderate might sound like no big deal, but they should always be treated.

When It's Not Sleep Apnea

It's a common scenario: a young woman with a normal BMI gets a sleep study and comes back with an AHI of zero. She didn't have sleep apnea, but she did have UARS (upper airway resistance syndrome). UARS is commonly overlooked, underdiagnosed, and not treated.

People with UARS can have an AHI of zero and still have many of the same symptoms of sleep apnea—sleepiness, anxiety, headaches, and fatigue to name a few. That's because AHI is calculated based on breathing interruptions that are 10 seconds or longer, and people with UARS often have breathing resistance or interruptions that are under nine seconds, but still have an impact.

The common UARS sufferer is not overweight, has low blood pressure, and has a healthy AHI—sometimes an AHI of zero. It's hard for their doctors to believe they still have sleep-disordered breathing that needs treatment. Even though people with UARS show up as healthy, non-snoring, thin 20-somethings with low blood pressure, they can turn into snoring women with OSA and high blood pressure by the time they're in their 40s and 50s.

Bottom line: sleep-disordered breathing is a spectrum. Sleep apnea is at the far right end of that spectrum. The key is to aggressively treat yourself when you're at the left or middle part of the spectrum so you *prevent* moving to the right of the spectrum.

Understanding the Location and the Cause

As good as the PSG is, there's one thing it won't tell you—and that's the exact location of the resistance or obstruction in your airway.

Sometimes the source of a more minor blockage is straightforward—like chronic allergies or a crooked passageway in the nose (called a deviated septum), and the treatments for those are also fairly straightforward.

But if you can breathe through your nose with ease, the obstruction that can cause sleep-disordered breathing is likely somewhere between the top of your airway (the back of the throat) and the bottom of your airway (the bottom of your neck). Knowing *where* the blockage is occurring is essential when choosing which treatment is right for you. Does your airway get blocked at the top, middle, or bottom of your throat? You have to address the entire airway, from the top of the throat to the bottom of the voice box.

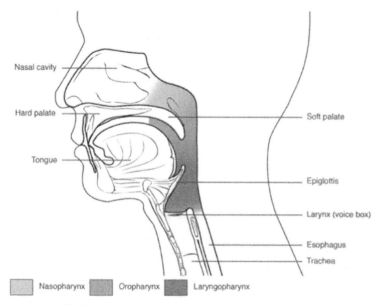

Find out where in your airway the resistance or constriction is located.

Airway Anatomy

Parts of the airway:

✓ Velopharynx (High)

✓ Oropharynx (Middle)

✓ Hypopharynx (Low)

Here's one way to find out where the obstruction is: ask your doctor for a Müller's Maneuver. A Müller's Maneuver is performed with a little camera that travels down the back of the throat to see what things look like back there.

Scuba divers and people who have trouble with pressure changes on planes learn to pop their ears by using the Valsalva maneuver—plugging their noses, closing their mouths, and trying to blow forcefully through their closed airways (like blowing up a balloon). This creates internal pressure that equalizes the pressure for your ears.

Müller's Maneuver is basically the same thing, only in reverse: you exhale and then close your airway and try hard to inhale. This creates negative pressure in your lungs, making them collapse. By watching closely what happens when you do this, your doctor can help determine the weak areas of your airway—and, therefore, possible causes of your sleep apnea.

Knowing not just what kind of sleep-disordered breathing you have, but also where and why the blockage is occurring, is essential. Keep that in mind in the next chapter, where we'll talk about all the different treatments for sleep-disordered breathing and how they work for different types of sleep breathing interruptions.

Chapter 5:
Step 2: Treat

I've always envied people who sleep easily. Their brains must be cleaner, the floorboards of the skull well swept, all the little monsters closed up in a steamer trunk at the foot of the bed.
— David Benioff, City of Thieves

So you've gotten your sleep test and perhaps a diagnosis from your sleep doctor. Now what?

No matter what, when you're treating your sleep-disordered breathing, your goals are to both:

1)   Be able to breathe through your nose with ease, and

2) Support your airway while your muscles are relaxed in deep sleep.

It's that simple. If you can keep the airway open, your body will take care of the rest.

Lifestyle and Bedroom Changes for Better Sleep Hygiene

Practicing good sleep hygiene is essential to quality sleep, but does not treat a collapsing airway. Do not look to these tips as the actual treatment for sleep-disordered breathing— follow these alongside your treatment.

➡ **Quit smoking.** Smoking can make sleep-disordered breathing symptoms worse by creating swelling in the upper airway.

➡ **Moderate alcohol.** Alcohol relaxes your throat muscles, causing you to snore and your airway to relax.

➡ **Watch your weight.** When you're overweight, the extra tissue in your neck may reposition the U-shaped bone in the neck that supports the tongue (the hyoid bone), narrowing your airway. The tongue can also expand along with your waistline. If this is the cause of your sleep apnea, losing weight may help the severity.

➡ **Manage allergies** through decongestants, nasal strips, or allergy-proofing your bedroom. Even the most perfect, wide-open airway is susceptible to swelling from allergies! (See Appendix A for tips on allergy-proofing your bedroom.)

➡ **Get a good pillow.** If you've been trained in CPR, you know that one of the first steps is to tilt the head back because it opens the airway. The same goes for when you're sleeping—a pillow that's good for the airway is one that either keeps you sleeping on your side with your spine in alignment or, on your back with your head slightly tilted back to open the airway. Tilting the head too far back constricts the airway.

A Review of Treatments

Positional Therapy

When you sleep on your back, gravity causes the jaw and tongue to fall back on the throat, making the airway more likely to collapse. When you sleep on your side, however, the jaw and tongue are less likely to fall back. For example, some people primarily have breathing resistance or interruptions while sleeping on their backs (thanks to gravity causing the jaw and tongue to fall back on the throat) but breathe normally while sleeping on their sides. In about 20% of people with obstructive sleep apnea, side sleeping reduces the number of interruptions to less than five, thanks to side sleeping's ability to significantly improve airway collapsibility.[38] In most cases, the minute you roll over, you reduce your number of disturbances. This may or may not apply to you and your airway—check if your sleep study recorded this and ask your sleep specialist if you exhibited "positional apneas" during the test.

Positional therapy can be used alone or together with another treatment. The device keeps you sleeping in the side position. Another option is to use a small device with "vibro-tactile feedback" technology. You wear it on the back of your neck. If you try to sleep on your back while wearing the device, it gently vibrates. This doesn't wake you up, but it does alert your body to change positions. But you don't even have to be this high tech.

---

38   Joosten SA, Edwards BA, Wellman A, Turton A, Skuza EM, Berger PJ, Hamilton GS. "The effect of body position on physiological factors that contribute to obstructive sleep apnea." *Sleep* 2015;38(9):1469−1478.

I've heard of people sleeping with tennis balls duct-taped to their shirts, and even full backpacks, which can work great!

Positional therapy can be used alone or together with another sleep apnea treatment.

CPAP and APAP Therapy

Most people aren't thrilled when their doctor recommends a CPAP machine. It can be pretty inconvenient when you just want to fall into bed—instead, you're hooking yourself up to a breathing machine. It might not be elegant, but here's why I like it:

- ✓ It has a long track record of efficacy and has the most evidence behind it.
- ✓ It's been around the longest, so it's often the easiest to get.
- ✓ It has a high success rate, if tolerated.
- ✓ It's the least invasive.
- ✓ It's the easiest to get insurance coverage for.
- ✓ It's a great back-up to have even if you have an oral appliance (discussed later), in case it gets lost, breaks, or if you need a back-up while you're having dental work done.

The CPAP is a machine that keeps your airway open while you sleep with the use of air pressure. CPAP stands for continuous positive airway pressure. The air comes through at a pre-set rate and keeps your airway open so that your breathing isn't interrupted, allowing you to access deep stage sleep. The mask you wear seals around your nose or both your nose and mouth. Positive pressure means that the air being blown down into your airway is enough to push back against the collapse of the muscles and tissues around the airway. It's the difference between a balloon that is deflated and a balloon that has form.

A CPAP machine has three parts:

1. Nasal pillows that fit inside the nose or a mask that fits over your nose or mouth, or both. Straps keep the mask in place.

2. A tube that connects the mask to the machine.

3. A motor in the machine that blows air into the tube.

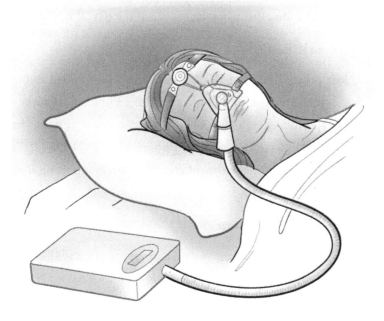

CPAP Tips

If you get a CPAP, the odds are against you: studies show that about 50% of people given a CPAP are forced to give it up

because they can't tolerate it—it makes them feel claustrophobic, they take off the mask during the night, or it leaves marks on the face to name a few of the most common issues. In the real world, adherence is actually closer to 20 to 30% since people are often given a CPAP without the training, support, and follow-up given to people in the studies.

Here's how you can beat the odds. The key thing to remember is that a CPAP is only effective for the nights that you actually wear it, so making it comfortable and becoming an expert are essential. For some, this will take time, but the payoff is huge.

Become an Expert

Most people are given a CPAP without being trained to use it. Insist that you get time with a CPAP technician, who can help you speed up the process of becoming an expert. Do not let the CPAP technician just send you home with it. Demand the education—it could make the difference between you using it or being forced to give up.

Make it Part of Your Routine

A CPAP isn't like a drug you take to knock out an infection. You'll have to adopt wearing and cleaning your CPAP as part of your daily routine. You'll also need to schedule follow-ups with your doctor once or twice a year to check in on the air pressure settings.

Get an Upgrade

The newest CPAP machines are as quiet as another person whispering in the same room, and are half the size of a shoebox. Upgrading to a newer model can often make it easier to sleep with, travel with, and keep in the bedroom.

Once you've been treated, are snoring less, and have reduced your AHI, you can look into getting an APAP, which is similar to the CPAP in that it applies positive pressure to the airway, but is a more modern and advanced machine that adapts to you.

An APAP (automatic positive airway pressure) machine adjusts the level of air it blows based on your needs during the night. The device has sensors that detect how well you are breathing at any given moment. The APAP constantly adjusts the air pressure according to this feedback. If you try to breathe but can't, it will increase the air pressure. If you're breathing fine, it will decrease the air pressure. It's a smarter CPAP.

The reason an APAP is a better solution is that it adapts to your changing needs as you heal. After sleeping with a CPAP for some time, the inflammation in the airway caused by snoring and airway resistance begins to decrease and the airway becomes less likely to collapse. If you lose weight, which is more likely after treating sleep-disordered breathing, you will need still less air pressure.

If you use the APAP together with a MAD, you'll likely need even less air since the MAD itself helps to keep the airway open. I'm a big fan of using a MAD in conjunction with an APAP, and consider this the gold standard for treating sleep-disordered breathing.

Join a Support Group

Getting healthy is always easiest when you do it with someone else, and it's no different when it comes to sleep. You're not alone, and finding a support group, whether in person or online, is one of the best ways to stick with it and have people who have been there before to give you advice or help you troubleshoot.

Get a Mask That Fits Perfectly

The key to comfort is a face mask that fits well. Don't hurry through this process. Really sit down and find a good mask provider. Test out several different masks until you find one that fits perfectly.

Make Sure You Can Breathe Through Your Nose

A CPAP can't deliver air to you effectively if your nose is stuffy. If you have to breathe through your mouth, you can get a full-face mask, but these are often harder to tolerate. Find out why you can't breathe through your nose and treat whatever condition is causing the problem.

Troubleshoot

Don't be afraid to tell your doctor if you're having a tough time tolerating the CPAP. Too many people think the CPAP is their only option and that "it's just the way it is," so they don't push back on the doctor, the doctor doesn't know there are problems, and the person ends up skipping the CPAP most nights because it's just unbearable. Follup up with your CPAP technician and work together on it.

Get Your Sleep Partner on Board

Sleeping hooked up to a mask certainly isn't sexy, but I encourage you to think of it this way: in most cases, snoring forces couples to sleep in separate bedrooms. Symptoms from sleep apnea often leave people too tired for sex, intimacy, and emotional connectedness. You need the CPAP to get through your day *and* have energy left over in the evenings to be with your partner. Lots of couples work around the CPAP and often find that it *improves* not just their sexual connection, but also their relationship as a whole.

Possible Positive Side Effects of CPAP and APAP:

- ✓ Bursts of energy (called "CPAP high") due to deep and restful sleep
- ✓ Improved mood
- ✓ Ability to focus and concentrate
- ✓ Improved academic or work performance
- ✓ Improved relationships with friends and loved ones

Possible Negative Side Effects:

- ✓ Irritation from noise or a mask that leaks air (blow-by)
- ✓ The constant pressure on your front teeth can cause them to shift and change your bite (how your teeth come together)

✓ Nasal congestion, headaches, bloating, dry eyes

✓ Increased risk of pneumonia

✓ Marks on the face upon waking

✓ Increase in cavities and swollen gums due to dry mouth

✓ Discomfort from mask or restricted movement

Don's CPAP Story

I was in my 40s. I didn't have as much energy as I used to, and I didn't understand why. The tiredness drove me to get a sleep study, where I found out I had an AHI of 22.

I was prescribed a CPAP. Immediately, my fatigue issues were solved. I love sleeping with the CPAP. I didn't have an adjustment period with it, except for having to remember to clean the thing! My one gripe is that I can't travel with it, and I travel a lot, whether it's for work or going on a camping trip. This is where I use my MAD, since it's travelproof.

Having a CPAP has changed my life so much that I want to make sure that my kids get the benefits of deep sleep earlier, unlike I did. We got my son Ben in for a sleep study, and he had an AHI of 6. We started treating him immediately.

Not everyone with sleep-disordered breathing or even sleep apnea will need a CPAP, but if you've gotten to a point where you're beyond mild sleep apnea, a CPAP can help give you back your life.

See the Resources section of this book for a list of in-person and online support groups for CPAP users, as well as what to do if you do not have insurance or cannot afford a CPAP. If you cannot tolerate a CPAP and want a MAD instead (which you'll read about next), see Appendix G for a form that will help you get coverage for your MAD.

Dental Appliances: MAD and TRD

There are two types of dental appliances you can get from your dentist: a mandibular advancement device (MAD) and tongue retaining device (TRD). Oral appliances can be used alone or in combination with other treatments.

If you do get a dental appliance, make sure you get it custom-made from your dentist. If you purchase an over-the-counter device online or from a drug store, be aware that *it could make the situation in your airway worse.* One-size-fits all devices aren't adjustable and aren't fitted by a professional who can ensure the device is moving you to the proper position. If you do choose a non-custom device, make sure you verify its efficacy following the instructions in Chapter 6 of this book.

MAD: Mandibular Advancement Device

A MAD (pronounced "mad") fits like a mouthguard or retainer. It helps keep the airway open by keeping the lower jaw jutting forward, which prevents the collapse of the tongue and soft tissues in the back of the throat. It also works by stabilizing the jaw while you're asleep.

The 8-Hour Sleep Paradox

The MAD:

- ✓ Repositions the lower jaw, tongue, and soft palate

- ✓ Stabilizes the lower jaw and tongue

- ✓ Increases the muscle tone of the tongue and flattens the tongue

Other names for the MAD:

- ✓ Sleep apnea device

- ✓ Herbst

- ✓ Oral appliance therapy (OAT)

Without MAD

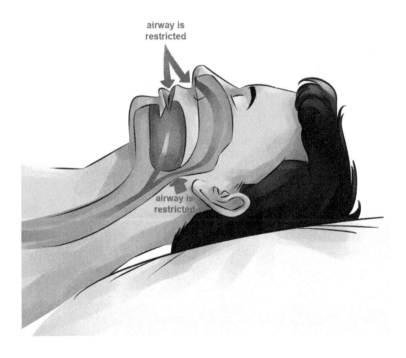

With MAD

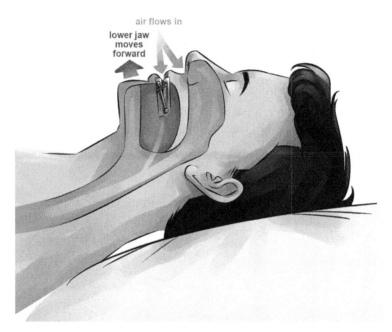

Advantages of MAD:

✓ No machine (CPAP) noise.

✓ Protects against and may prevent grinding (bruxism).

✓ Small and convenient to carry while traveling and doesn't require electricity.

✓ Virtually reversible and non-invasive.

✓ Can drink water with it, take medication, or speak to your bed partner.

✓ Less likely to be accidentally removed in the middle of the night.

✓ Sexier than a CPAP mask.

✓ May fix TMD (but can cause some jaw pain, especially as you're getting used to wearing it for the first time). Some doctors and dentists may tell you that you shouldn't use a MAD if you have jaw pain or TMD (temporomandibular joint disorder), but many times the root cause of TMD can be years of grinding due to a small airway. Opening up the airway stops the impulse to grind, and eventually the TMD and facial pain.

✓ Acts as a retainer to keep your teeth straight.

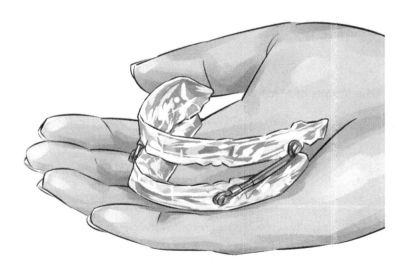

A mandibular advancement device, or MAD (pronounced "mad")

Drawbacks to MAD:

✓ Can take a few weeks or months to get used to wearing it.

✓ Can change your bite over time (not always a bad thing).[39]

✓ Doesn't pull the tongue forward for a small number of people.

✓ Hard to find a dentist that has experience in this area. (See the Resources section of this book for help with this.)

✓ Drooling (which is temporary).

✓ Doesn't work well if you have a high BMI or severe sleep apnea.

Getting Your New MAD: What to Expect

When you first try on your MAD, it can be uncomfortable, just like a new retainer or wearing Invisalign or braces for the first time.

Tips for Comfort:

✓ *Make sure that your MAD is not too thick.* If you feel like you're being opened up too far, that could close your airway. Make sure your teeth come pretty close together, if not all the way together, at rest.

---

39   The original use of the MAD was as an orthodontic appliance to help people with overbites. In many cases, a MAD can actually improve the bite, which is how the teeth come together. For people with a Class II bite (overbite) 90% of people experience an improvement in their bite aftering wearing the MAD. In people with a Class III bite (underbite) only 50% of people had a change in their bite. My thought on the bite changing is that it's trivial compared to sleep quality. Changes in bite can be dealt with, but a lack of deep sleep is unacceptable. If a MAD is your best option, bite changes are something you can live with and manage with your dentist.

✓ *It can take several months to get used to the MAD,* especially if you grind and clench, carry your stress in your neck and jaw, or drink caffeine. It's normal if you have pain in the beginning that gets better each night as your jaw gets used to letting go and letting the MAD move you forward. But if you have pain after wearing the MAD that gets worse every time you wear it, call your dentist right away. Your dentist will check and adjust the device at several appointments to make sure the device fits properly.

✓ *Take it slow.* MADs are adjustable, and your dentist will work with you to calibrate it—meaning, adjust it forward and backward until you find the level of advancement that feels right and opens the airway the right amount. Start at only 50 or 60% of the full advancement so your jaw can get used to it before advancing further.

Your MAD should come with something called a *morning repositioner,* which is a small retainer-like device you wear in the morning while your jaw returns from the forward position to its normal position.

The best way to use the morning repositioner is to pop it in once you take out your MAD in the morning and wear it while you apply makeup, cook breakfast, or get ready for the day.

A lot of people find that they can skip the morning repositioner if they sit on the toilet in the morning in the "thinker pose," putting pressure on their jaw to push it back. Within minutes, the jaw is back to normal. After some time, usually a year, the transition back to your normal bite (how your teeth come together) every morning is almost immediate.

By the way, dogs love chewing the morning repositioner, so be careful not to leave it where your dog can grab it!

The MAD Routine

→ Leave the MAD on the nightstand while you read or go through your bedtime routine, and then pop it in your mouth before shutting out the lights.

→ In the morning, pop out the MAD and leave it soaking in water and baking soda all day. Always keep it moist.

→ Wear the morning repositioner while in the shower or cooking breakfast.

→ Repeat.

→ Bring your MAD with you to every teeth cleaning appointment.

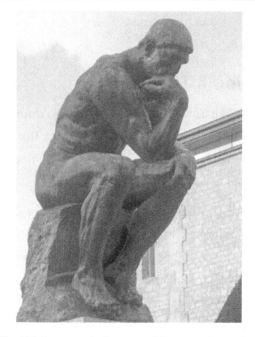

The thinker pose helps reposition your lower jaw after sleeping with your MAD.

Which MAD is Best?

Here's a counterintuitive tip I give to people trying to figure out if the device their dentist recommends is a good one: go with a MAD that's on the Medicare-approved list of MADs. Why? Medicare looks into the data and research behind each appliance before approving it, because Medicare doesn't want to pay out for anything that isn't 100% proven. It's hard to make it onto the list, and there will be some MADs that should be on the list that aren't yet—but it's a good rule of thumb to go by if you're faced with a decision and want a guarantee that the MAD you choose is clinically proven to be effective.

Check to see the complete list of MADs approved by Medicare in Appendix B.

Calibration & Titration

If you get a CPAP or a MAD, you'll need to go through a process called titration (for the CPAP) or calibration (for the MAD), which is essentially tweaking the device until you find the optimal setting for you.

With a CPAP, titration is done during a sleep study via trial and error. The sleep technician will adjust the air pressure of the CPAP and see how you respond to find where the optimal setting is. With a MAD, calibration is done by your dentist over the course of multiple dental visits to find the optimal position for the jaw to open the airway. Calibration of a MAD can also be done during a sleep study with a motorized MAD that is moved forward and backward on the fly by the sleep technician to find the position where the airway responds best. No device is one-size-fits-all and titration and calibration are essential to find the right setting for you and your airway.

TRD: Tongue Retaining Device

A TRD is a soft plastic bulb that you squeeze and then insert your tongue into. Squeezing the bulb creates suction, which pulls your tongue forward and holds onto it. Held forward like this, the tongue is unable to fall back into the mouth during deep sleep— which means it can't block your airway. They come in small, medium, or large, and are only available through a dentist.

A TRD pulls the tongue forward, but not the jaw, which is why it's not as reliable as a mandibular advancement device. A TRD stretches the tongue forward, whereas a MAD takes the base of the tongue and pulls it away from the airway, which is why the TRD is not the go-to device for mandibular advancement. An advantage is that it can provide immediate benefit, doesn't require any adjustments, may have less of an effect on your bite, and is the least expensive treatment for someone without any insurance (around $300 to $500 from your dentist). The TRD shouldn't be used on people with nasal obstruction.[40]

---

40   Diane S. Lazard, Marc Blumen, Pierre Lévy, Pierre Chauvin, Dorothée Fragny, Isabelle Buchet, and Frédéric Chabolle, "The Tongue-Retaining Device: Efficacy and Side Effects in Obstructive Sleep Apnea Syndrome," *Journal of Clinical Sleep Medicine* 5, no. 5 (2009): 431-438, *http://www.ncbi.nlm.nih.gov/pmc/articles/PMC2762714/*

Tongue Exercises and Myofunctional Therapy

The research shows that a physical therapy called myofunctional therapy may reduce symptoms of sleep-disordered breathing and improve (but not cure) mild to moderate OSA. When these muscles are retrained out of habits we form from childhood, obstruction to the airway can be decreased.

Take a look at the tongue exercises included in Appendix F and consider consulting with a myofunctional therapist. I use the Academy of Orofacial Myofunctional Therapy's "Find a Therapist Near You" web page when referring my own patients: *http://aomtinfo.org/find-a-therapist-2.*

Surgery

There are straightforward types of surgeries, such as removing tonsils or adenoids in children or fixing a deviated septum. These surgeries, when recommended by a specialist, should almost always be done. They almost always work, because the anatomical cause of the breathing difficulty is clearly understood and the methodology during the surgery is targeted. Risk is low.

Other surgeries, where there is no clear anatomical obstruction, are significantly more complicated. Once we get into this territory, things are not as clear, and the results are much more unpredictable. This is where surgery becomes as much an art as a science. You absolutely need to be in the hands of someone who really knows what he or she is doing—ideally, someone who does only this kind of surgery, all day long, and is a true specialist.

Drive or fly if you have to get in to get to a university with a large sleep clinic that specializes in these types of surgeries.

Surgery was the go-to decades ago, but things have changed. The formerly popular UPPP surgery has been criticized for being only 50% effective after the first year of surgery and for causing things to get worse thanks to scar tissue buildup. We now know that non-surgical methods should be attempted first. Besides, the UPPP is quite an uncomfortable and painful surgery. Having said that, in some cases, if the surgery is tailored specifically to a person's anatomical issues and unique airway, it can be a good option. As risky as surgery is, it's not nearly as risky as living with untreated sleep-disordered breathing.

Here's what you need to consider if you're thinking about surgery:

✓ Surgery can improve sleep apnea and sleep-disordered breathing.

✓ Fully understand the complications and the risk that surgery could make things worse.

✓ Make sure you have realistic expectations. The first part of a good surgery is making sure that the surgery is appropriate and necessary.

What makes a surgery successful in treating sleep apnea:

✓ If the surgery reduces AHI by 50% (for example, from an AHI of 80 to 40).

✓ If the surgery reduces AHI to less than 5, it is considered a cure, but this is rare and difficult to do with surgery, so discuss your unique situation with your surgeon and do your homework.

My recommendations:

✓ The key to a good surgery is identifying something in the body where, if you modify it, there will be some benefit—and that's not always a given, so discuss this with your doctor.

✓ Don't be swayed by fancy instruments, lasers, or the latest technology in surgical tools—go purely based on the skill and reputation of your surgeon and how many surgeries s/he has done.

✓ Discuss with your doctor or surgeon about what s/he considers success.

Don't take it lightly.

Common Surgeries for Sleep Apnea:

✓ Nasal surgery: Cartilage in the nose that is off-center and impedes breathing (deviated septum) is corrected to allow for proper breathing. (Discussed in detail on the next page.)

✓ Tonsils or adenoid removal: Improves space at the back of the throat by removing common airway obstructions in children—the tonsils and adenoids.

✓ Uvulopalatopharyngoplasty (UPPP or UP3): Involves soft tissue removal on the back of the throat and roof of the mouth, increasing the airway's width at the entrance to the throat.

✓ Mandibular maxillary advancement surgery: Corrects a small lower jaw with an overbite to improve space at the back of the throat.

Nasal Surgery for Deviated Septum (Septoplasty)

All of us have bone and cartilage that divide the insides of our noses in half. In about 80% of the population, this "wall" is off-center, or crooked, which can impact sleep breathing. This is called a deviated septum, and it's diagnosed by an ear, nose, and throat doctor (ENT) who will examine the inside of your nose to make the diagnosis.

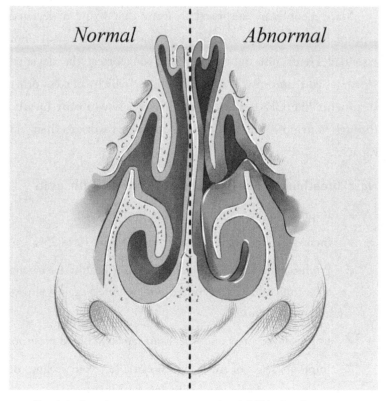

Deviated septums are common—about 80% of us have one. It's a condition that often goes unnoticed, but its impact on sleep and health can be debilitating.

Symptoms of a deviated septum include:

✓ Nosebleeds

✓ Loud breathing or snoring during sleep

✓ Postnasal drip

✓ Nasal congestion or stuffy nose

✓ Inability to breathe through one nostril

Many people are surprised to learn that fixing a deviated septum isn't typically a cure-all. But that doesn't mean it's not essential! Here's how it works: when you correct the deviated septum, you improve nasal breathing, which makes other treatments like CPAP and MAD effective. If you can't breathe through your nose, any other treatments won't work to their full capacity.

Nasal breathing is an essential part of good health, as it:

✓ Improves carbon dioxide levels in the body.

✓ Increases oxygen absorption by the lungs by 10 to 25%.

✓ Produces nitric oxide, which keeps you healthy by having an antimicrobial effect and helping to protect against viruses and other germs.

✓ Improves the stress response, heart rate, and blood pressure.

✓ Improves sense of smell, which can affect your feelings of "fullness" and help you maintain a healthy weight.

✓ Promotes good facial growth and straight teeth in a developing child.

✓ Could have beneficial effects on the microbiome, which is the vast array of microbes in our bodies responsible for biological processes involved with immunity, memory, heart health, mental health and brain health, and maintaining a healthy weight.

A lot of people don't realize their nose is stuffy because *they're so used to it.* We don't pay attention to how we breathe, so it's all normal to us. You can have your nasal breathing verified by your doctor or dentist.

The Best Treatment for You

I'm asked almost daily, "Well, what's the best treatment? I'll just go with that." My answer to this question is three-part:

1. Consider where the obstruction is.

2. The best treatment is the one you use.

3. Don't choose just one!

1. Where's the Obstruction?

Remember that it's essential to know the *location* of the obstruction or resistance in your airway—is it in the upper, middle, or lower part of the airway? In the last chapter, we talked about a Müller's Maneuver, which tells your doctor where in your airway the obstruction or resistance might be.

If your blockage is at the bottom of your airway, opening up the top of the airway by pulling the tongue forward (with a MAD) isn't going to work. If you give a CPAP or a MAD to someone who is suffering from a deviated septum or chronic allergies, being unable to breathe through their nose is going to block a lot of the good that a CPAP or MAD can do. A common misconception is that nasal strips can open the airway and stop snoring, but all they do is open the entrance to a constricted airway, having no effect on the constriction further down the airway.

Bottom line: some treatments are great for upper airway resistance. Others are better for obstructions deeper down in the airway. A Müller's Maneuver—not a PSG—tells you where the blockage or resistance is located so that you can pick the right treatment.

2. Effectiveness vs. Using It

If you don't like the first treatment your doctor prescribes, you have options. Proving a treatment is effective in a clinical study is one thing—actually using it yourself in the real world is quite another. "Compliance" is the word sleep specialists use to describe whether you're using your treatment, and it's an important concept when you consider that 50% of people given a CPAP *cannot or do not use it.* The most effective treatment in the world isn't going to cure your sleep-disordered breathing unless you use it.

People feel guilty about this, but the truth is, we doctors need to be better about supporting our patients and understanding that what works in a clinical study doesn't always work in real life. This is a lifestyle change—a big one. Give it an honest shot, but trust your gut when it's time to move on and try something else.

If the first treatment your doctor gives you is not working, try, try again. No matter what the statistics and the research and the experts tell you, you have to try alternatives if something isn't working. Ask to try something else. Something that's less than optimal that's used on a regular basis is better than something that's optimal that's not used!

- ✓ If a CPAP feels too blowy, try adding a MAD, which can open up your airway to make the CPAP more comfortable.

- ✓ If a MAD hurts your jaw, stop wearing it for a few weeks, and start again in a less advanced position and calibrate it more slowly. In the meantime, wear your CPAP.

- ✓ If a TRD wakes you up because you can't breathe through your nose, try a MAD, which will let you breathe through your mouth while you treat your nasal obstruction.

- ✓ If you feel like you've tried everything and nothing seems to feel right to you, look into surgical options.

This is like trying several different keys before finding out which one unlocks the door—you'll know it when it's right. Trust your gut and don't give up. The medical community is just beginning to understand that much of the time, two treatments used together are what it takes to unlock that door.

Am I a Good Candidate for a MAD?

When discussing your PSG results with your sleep doctor and dentist, here are some indications that you are a good candidate for MAD therapy:

1. If you had a CPAP titration study, look at the pressure used that night that gave you the right amount of pressure to keep your airway from collapsing and prevented you from waking up. The higher the pressure, the more difficult it will be for a MAD to achieve efficacy.

2. If your AHI was lower when sleeping on your side as opposed to sleeping on your back, this is an indication that you are likely a good candidate.

3. If you have more hypopneas (slow or shallow breathing) than apneas (a breathing pause lasting 10 or more seconds), you are likely a good candidate.

4. If your oxygen desaturation percentage is unusually high when compared to your AHI, chances are you will respond well to MAD therapy.

5. If you have a high AHI but are thin, this is a good sign that MAD therapy will work well. My wife Roseann had severe obstructive sleep apnea but because her BMI was low, she responded very well to MAD therapy.

6. Look at how long the apneas are. If they are just over 10 seconds, no matter how many, it means that it doesn't take much to reopen the airway. The MAD has a high likelihood of success if this is the case. Longer apneas indicate that it takes more effort to open the airway, and the MAD may only be partially effective.

---

3. Combination Therapy

Combination therapy is exactly what it sounds like—a combination of two treatments working together.

Some of the more common combination therapies I've seen:

✓ Sleeping on your side (positional therapy) with a MAD.

✓ Wearing a MAD and APAP together. (This works tremendously well for lots of people. I think this could be a new gold standard in the future as more research is done on combination treatments.)[41]

✓ Nasal surgery to breathe better through your nose combined with CPAP.

✓ Several months of myofunctional therapy and tongue exercises combined with a MAD.

✓ Mouth taping while wearing a MAD or CPAP.

Don't get locked into thinking you have to be stuck with one method! I've had numerous patients who dislike two treatments separately but love them together.

One of those patients was Karen, a petite, 75-year-old woman who was slightly overweight and had an AHI of almost 80. She was optimistic and cheerful, which I think may have made her path to diagnosis much slower. She tried the CPAP but, after many months of trying to make it work, decided that she would rather deal with the consequences of untreated sleep apnea.

Her nephew, a Silicon Valley CEO, also came to see me around the same time for a MAD. He flat-out refused to get a sleep study. "I don't have time; I just need to start sleeping better," he insisted. So we made him the device, and of course, he started to feel much better. It wasn't long before he told his aunt about his experience.

---

41   Olivier M. Vanderveken, "Combination Therapy for Obstructive Sleep Apnea in Order to Achieve Complete Disease Alleviation: from Taboo to New Standard of Care?" *Journal of Dental Sleep Medicine* 2, no. 3 (2015): 7-8, http://dx.doi.org/10.15331/jdsm.4428.

So she came into my office telling me she wanted the MAD. I was concerned that a MAD wouldn't be enough for her severe sleep apnea, so I and her sleep specialist kept pushing the CPAP. We reached a stalemate with me telling her that she couldn't have a MAD, and her insisting she'd rather die than use a CPAP. Dramatic, I know!

Finally, I made a deal with her. I explained how dangerous it was for her not to wear her CPAP with an AHI that was so severe. I told her I would make her a MAD knowing it would not cure her sleep apnea and that she should be wearing her CPAP, only to see how much we could reduce her AHI. I didn't mention that I was going to try to convince her to wear the CPAP again.

With the MAD, we got Karen's AHI down to 19—still moderate sleep apnea, but at least no longer severe. She began feeling much better and told me she was cured, and I told her she wasn't; there was still more to go.

Over many visits to help calibrate the MAD, I told her about a new device that was like a CPAP but newer and smarter—the APAP. In the end, I convinced her to try it.

When Karen wore her APAP and MAD together, her sleep study showed she had an AHI of well under five. What made me happy wasn't just the AHI—it was that we had found a way for her to have perfect *compliance* with her treatment, which as we've discussed is just as important as the *efficacy* of the treatment. I don't just want a treatment that works for my patients; I want one that they also want to use.

Combination therapy saved Karen's life. The lesson here: find a team that's willing to work with you.

The Importance of the Right Team

If you have a hammer, everything looks like a nail. Your dentist will want to give you an oral appliance. Your surgeon will want to do surgery. Your sleep specialist will want to give you a CPAP. That's not to say any of these things are wrong, but having the right team of specialists working together on your behalf means you'll get to the correct end point more quickly.

Also be aware that the only specialist qualified to *diagnose* sleep-disordered breathing is a sleep specialist MD. Your general practitioner doctor or dentist is not allowed to give you that diagnosis, although they may strongly suggest you go get diagnosed based on what they're seeing in you. It is out of scope for anyone other than an MD who *also specializes in sleep medicine* to give you the diagnosis. As for treatment, there are lots of different practitioners and therapists who can help you.

Who Does What

I've added this simple chart as a reference guide to help you understand who can help you with what in your quest to diagnose and treat your sleep-disordered breathing.

Who Does What on Your Sleep Team

Specialist	Screen and Refer	Measure	Treat	Verify
General practitioner (MD)	X			
Sleep specialist (MD)		X	X	X
ENT specializing in sleep (MD)		X	X	X
Sleep medicine dentist (DDS)	X		X	
Myofunctional therapist (RDH)			X	
Buteyko breathing instructor			X	
CPAP technician			X	

Some Early Indications That Your Treatment Is Working

➡ You wake up with no memory of the time between when you fell asleep and when you woke up.

➡ You don't get up to go to the bathroom in the middle of the night.

➡ You wake up before the alarm goes off and you think it's earlier than it really is. This is what I refer to as "amnesiac sleep" and it means you were in deep sleep.

➡ You wake up feeling refreshed and you don't feel like hitting the snooze button.

➡ Your body wakes you up earlier than usual and you are suddenly wide-awake.

➡ You tend to go to bed earlier and on a more regular schedule, not because you're tired, but because you're actually enjoying sleep more and subconsciously looking forward to it.

➡ Food portion control becomes easier.

➡ You feel more alert during the day and become more articulate in your daily conversations.

➡ You find it easier to focus and be creative.

→ You find yourself feeling happier, less anxious, and more patient with life's daily challenges.

→ Your joints hurt less.

→ You lose weight naturally without dieting or exercise.

→ You don't experience the afternoon slump as often and your energy stays more consistent throughout the day.

→ Your morning headaches go away.

→ Your jaw pain has improved or gone away, your mouth is less dry, and it's much easier to open your mouth wide at the dentist or during a meal.

→ You no longer fall asleep while watching TV.

→ You have more courage and mental stamina.

If putting together a sleep team seems like a lot of work, think of it this way: Your chances of becoming ill or dying from a complication of sleep-disordered breathing are higher than many common cancers. Cancer treatment centers have teams of different specialists, therapists, and social workers who work together to care for patients. As typical with the modern healthcare system, we're better organized when it comes to late-stage diseases, rather than early-stage symptoms and prevention. Creating this team for your own sleep-disordered breathing is essential to get the best result.

Chapter 6:
Step 3: Verify

Sleep is closing your eyes and trusting you will heal.
—Danielle Barone

When Karen came in to see me six months after she started using her MAD (mandibular advancement device), she was elated. She was feeling so much better. Her GERD (gastroesophageal reflux disease) had gone away, she had halved her depression medication, and she was staying up until 10 or 11 p.m. and waking up at 6 a.m. without any trouble. Her grandkids, whom I also see in my practice, actually *complained* that she had so much energy.

"That's great," I explained to Karen, "but we don't know how well you're really sleeping. We've got to send you back for a *split study*."

A split study is a PSG where the sleep technician and doctor work with you throughout the night, adjusting your CPAP, MAD, or other treatment to find the best solution for you to keep your airway open. If your first PSG was to diagnose your degree of sleep-disordered breathing, then the split study is an additional PSG to determine how effective your treatment is. Just because you've been given a solution doesn't mean that you have achieved efficacy. Split studies verify that your treatment has been calibrated for your unique situation.

We had adjusted Karen's MAD to almost 100% of her jaw's maximum forward position, and she said she felt great and thanked me profusely. After she got her split study, we saw her AHI had dropped—from 25 to nine—but we still had room to improve. In fact, over the course of the next few months and after a second split study, we were able to get her AHI to drop to zero—but only because she went back to verify her treatment and her sleep team was able to work together on her behalf. Had she not verified, she would have felt she was sleeping well, but her AHI would have still been at nine—still on the continuum of disease.

It's far too common that someone who is given treatment for sleep-disordered breathing immediately starts to feel better and stops there. The problem with this is, most treatments might improve your sleep-disordered breathing right away by moving you left on the continuum, but they won't improve it fully, all the way to the left. Furthermore, we tend to be overly optimistic when it comes to medical treatment. We think, "Oh, I'm not snoring anymore!" and think we're cured—but feeling better doesn't necessarily mean you don't have more room to improve. Scientific verification is the key to knowing that, for the rest of your life, you will obtain optimal sleep.

Verifying is perhaps the most essential step, but it's also the most frequently skipped step. It's an easy one to skip—you start sleeping with your CPAP or MAD, or you have a surgery done, and you start to feel better. When we feel better, we're much less likely to go back to the doctor. Most people want to skip verification because they feel better, but also, some doctors and dentists don't emphasize it enough.

Imagine the difference between these two scenarios: just feeling better with treatment *or* scientifically verifying that your treatment is indeed keeping your airway open at night. Just having the peace of mind that you've calibrated your treatment all the way will make you sleep better in itself!

How to Verify Your Sleep Ability

All that "verify" means is that you have to go in for a split study, which is a PSG for one night that compares half the night sleeping *without* treatment to the rest of the night sleeping *with* treatment.

This is something you may have to push for. The gold standard for verification is a PSG, for the same reason a PSG is the gold standard for diagnosing sleep-disordered breathing. Do all that you can to get a PSG, instead of one of the simpler tests, which may give you a false sense of security by underreporting on the severity of your sleep-disordered breathing—making your treatment look more effective than it actually is.

Successful verification doesn't happen just once or even twice. It will happen for the rest of your life. That's because sleep ability doesn't stay the same—just like weight or cholesterol, it is constantly changing, and you have to keep measuring to make sure you notice those changes and change your treatment accordingly. How do you verify your weight? You hop on the scale. There's no way to do that with sleep, except to go in for a PSG.

Sleep ability gets worse for everyone as we get older—even if you don't gain weight—because the airway muscles lose their tone with age. Sleep ability also gets worse with life events such as menopause or pregnancy. Getting medical treatment or taking a new drug can impact the airway as well.

Factors that can change your sleep ability

- ➡ Getting older
- ➡ Weight fluctuations
- ➡ Hormonal fluctuations
- ➡ Pregnancy
- ➡ Menopause
- ➡ Allergies

When and How Often Should I Verify?

This is something you and your sleep specialist have to discuss given your specific condition. For example, if you have the comorbidities of sleep apnea—heart disease, stroke, high blood pressure, diabetes—you'll want to verify more often. If you're further left on the spectrum—UARS, mild sleep apnea, or snoring due to weight gain from pregnancy, for example—you might need to verify less often. This is an important conversation to have with your sleep physician. Don't assume that your sleep doctor or CPAP supplier will contact you for follow-ups; mark your calendar with a recall schedule or reminders to make follow-up appointments.

Even if you're feeling great and don't have any symptoms, it doesn't hurt to check in regularly in between PSGs. Check in with your sleep partner, use a sleep app that records the noises you make during sleep, or see if your activity tracking device reports back any changes.

People verify their exercise and diet by measuring blood pressure or weight. We verify our health by measuring HDL, LDL and triglycerides for heart disease. Why wouldn't you verify your sleep? You've put this much effort into getting through steps one and two—it would be shortchanging yourself if you didn't at least verify that all your effort was actually working. Lifelong verification is the difference between a false sense of security and true wellness.

Chapter 7:
Insurance Tips & Tricks:
How to Get Coverage for a MAD

First, I had time, but no money;
then I had money, but no time.
Finally, I had time and money,
but no health to make use of my wealth.
—RVM Foundation

There's a need for accepting responsibility—for a person's life and
making choices that are not just ones for immediate, short-term
comfort. You need to make an investment, and the investment is in
health and education.
—Buzz Aldrin

Insurance coverage for just about every sleep-disordered breathing treatment is fairly straightforward—unless you're considering a MAD. The good news is that most people's medical insurance has partial to full coverage for MADs. But you will need to know some of the ins and outs of how to get yours covered.

Your dentist's office may or may not help you maximize your medical insurance, but if it doesn't, don't worry—you aren't stuck! With a little self-education and a lot of advocating, you can get the coverage you need.

Here's what you'll need to know.

Medical, Not Dental, Insurance Covers Oral Appliances

Sleep apnea is diagnosed by an MD, not a dentist, so dental insurance companies do not cover oral appliances. Even though a MAD will be made by your dentist, coverage is in the realm of medical, not dental, insurance.

You Don't Have to Have Sleep Apnea to Get Coverage

In some cases, your sleep study might show that you have a low average AHI; however, if you look at specific moments during the test, you might see that you have severe apneas at certain points during the night. Your average AHI can easily be brought down by some long stretches of low AHIs. Ask your sleep specialist physician for his or her help in picking these moments of more severe apnea, despite a lower overall AHI, to help you get insurance coverage.

Don't Leave Anything Out of Your Health History

If you have a mild diagnosis, such as UARS, snoring, or mild sleep apnea, it is typically harder to get coverage than a diagnosis of, say, moderate sleep apnea. Insurance companies will sometimes not provide coverage unless there is hypertension, insomnia, excessive daytime sleepiness, or other late-stage diseases associated with sleep apnea. In other words, you have to be sick for the insurance companies to pay. This is why it is up to you to make sure that you are very specific in describing your symptoms to your doctor.

Be Involved with the Process

One great way to get involved is to print out your insurance claim form and bring it in with you to your dental appointments. Your dental office might not have medical insurance forms available, but your insurance company's website should. By bringing in the form in person, you can expedite the insurance process.

What You'll Need to Give Your Insurance Provider[42]

Get a Referral from Your Primary Care Physician

Many medical insurance plans require you to have a referral to your sleep medicine specialist on file. This should be as simple as a quick phone call to your primary care doctor explaining what you need.

Get a Sleep Apnea Diagnosis from a Specialist

Your dentist can screen for sleep apnea and provide you with a MAD, but your dentist cannot diagnose sleep apnea or sleep-disordered breathing. This is important because medical insurance plans *require a diagnosis from a sleep specialist who is a physician*, such as an ENT or a sleep specialist. This specialist also needs to prescribe a MAD to you.

Make sure to:

✓ Get a written diagnosis of sleep-disordered breathing from the MD on file.

✓ Get a letter from that MD recommending a MAD.

---

42   For more information, check out this handy FAQ from the American Academy of Dental Sleep Medicine: *http://www.aadsm.org/Resources/pdf/FAQInsuranceReimbursement.pdf.*
This resource may also be helpful: *http://blog.sleepfoundation.org/dental-devices-for-sleep-apnea-are-covered-by-insurance.*
If you need an oral appliance, I also recommend this resource, which has a chart of codes used by insurance companies: *http://www.dentaleconomics.com/articles/print/volume-103/issue-5/features/you-can-do-it-oral-sleep-apnea-therapy-coded-correctly.html.*

Fill Out a Compliance History Form

Some insurance companies require a formal letter to confirm that you can't use a CPAP, and therefore, require a MAD. See Appendix G for the form written by insurance companies that shows that you're unable to use a CPAP effectively, which may help you get coverage for your MAD. Include that form in the things you give your insurance company.

If you fill out this form, you're more likely to get your MAD covered. This form is another reason to start with a CPAP. When the insurance company has a record on file that you tried CPAP and were intolerant, they can justify covering a MAD for you.

Provide a Recent Sleep Study

Your insurance company will need a copy of your sleep study, so make sure to have it available. Make sure it's also a recent study; many insurance companies may deny your claim if you file with a sleep study that isn't recent.

Know What Language to Use

The MAD is sometimes a complicated one for insurance companies because it's treatment coming from a dentist, with a diagnosis from a physician—so it's paid for by medical, not dental insurance. Hang in there! If the first person you speak to on the phone gives you a no, ask to speak to a supervisor or manager.

You may have to explain to your insurance provider what a MAD is and why you need it—both over the phone and in your forms. The phrase I've found most helpful for getting claims through is: "custom fabricated oral device used to reduce upper airway collapsibility." You can also give the person on the phone "Code E0486" which is the code used for the MAD.

Keep in mind that, for many insurance companies, it's standard practice to reject claims the first time; it makes things easier and cheaper for them if people give up easily. So make sure they know you aren't the sort of person who'll give up!

Find Out If Your Insurance Company Requires Authorization

Some medical insurance companies require authorization before you begin treatment. If this is the case, be sure to get authorization from your insurance company before you begin treatment. If you don't, you could get denied. Know your policy!

How to Choose a MAD That Will Get Approved

There are hundreds of different MADs out there, and not all of them are approved by insurance. If you go with a MAD that's *not* on the Medicare-approved list—whether or not you have Medicare—chances are, it will not be approved by insurance.

As of January 4, 2013, these are the only devices that are eligible for Medicare reimbursement:[43]

- ✓ Herbst by Dynaflex
- ✓ Herbst by Gergen's Orthodontic Lab
- ✓ TAP by Airway Management
- ✓ TAP 3 Elite by Airway Management
- ✓ Telescopic Herbst by Great Lakes Orthodontics
- ✓ SUAD by Strong Dental LTD
- ✓ SUAD Elite by Strong Dental LTD
- ✓ UCLA Modified Herbst by Space Maintainers Laboratory

What to Know If You Have Medicare

If you have Medicare, you'll want to see a Medicare sleep dentist. Medicare will only provide you with coverage if you see a sleep dentist who's on the Medicare plan.

The code that Medicare uses for oral appliances is called "durable medical equipment," which is the same code category for the CPAP.

Medicare covers 80% of the cost of your oral appliance, along with a deductible of $160.

Be certain that your MAD is on the list of Medicare-approved oral appliances (see Appendix B). If it isn't, it won't be eligible for coverage.

---

43   "Medicare PDAC Verifies More Devices," *American Academy of Dental Sleep Medicine*, 2013, *http://www.aadsm.org/articles.aspx?id=3565.*

If Your Insurance Claim is Denied, You Have Options

If your insurance claim is denied, you can request a peer-to-peer review. In this review, your dentist can review your situation with your physician to explain why he or she recommends MAD therapy. You'll still need a diagnosis from a sleep specialist physician in order for this to be successful.

Don't take "no" as an answer. For Medicare and for many private insurance companies, applying, getting turned down, and then appealing is standard procedure. Expect that you may get denied the first time and be ready to appeal the decision.

Above all, remember this: insurance should never stop you from getting proper treatment. The cost of diagnosing and treating sleep-disordered breathing can be significant, often over $3,000. If you are uninsured or underinsured, or simply don't have a lot of free time, it can be easy to slip into inaction. Remember this, though: deciding not to treat sleep-disordered breathing now isn't choosing the cheaper option or saving you time, because the consequences of untreated sleep-disordered breathing are much more costly and will take up more of your time, eat into your productivity, or even shorten your life in the long run. In this way, early diagnosis and treatment are always worth it.

Epilogue:
What It's Like to Wake Up

Sleep is the most important part of recovery.
—Unknown

My Story

You might be wondering how my story ends.

My PSG sleep study revealed that I had an AHI of 12 and my doctor told me I was fine. That might have been the end of it save for my wife's severe sleep apnea. As she was being treated, I read over a hundred sleep studies and learned everything I could about sleep apnea. Then I looked again at my test results.

"Fine," the doctor had told me. I wasn't fine.

I read my sleep study again, and now I knew what I was looking at. I was shocked to find that my oxygen saturation levels were dipping as low as 83% at times (95% is normal), which meant that my brain was suffocating from lack of oxygen every night. I had sleep apnea, and I needed treatment.

I started treating myself. Before long, I was able to get my AHI down to zero by sleeping with a MAD. I verify that my AHI stays at zero with a PSG every few years. I could not have written this book with an AHI of 12. I wouldn't even have considered it.

Knowledge Can Save Your Life

In my younger years, I used to try to get by with as little sleep as possible. I used to be a night owl. Now I look forward to sleeping each night. I sleep deeply. I experience amnesiac sleep. I wake up alert, refreshed, and healed. I face each morning without dread, grogginess, or alarm. My temper is more even, my mind sharper, my future brighter.

After getting treated, my patients are happier, healthier, sharper, more articulate. They become better spouses, parents, and friends. One of my patients said treatment gave her the courage to finally get out of a dysfunctional relationship. Another says sleeping better gave her the energy to pursue a life-long dream of starting a business. One father said treatment gave him back evenings with his kids. One young woman who almost could not finish high school said treatment was what got her to community college, then on to earn her bachelor's degree, and finally reached her ultimate goal of graduate school in one of the top programs in the nation. There are so many more stories just like these. Waking up is not an insignificant event. This is where my story ends, but where yours begins. What would waking up look like for you if you could breathe better and get more deep sleep?

I'd like to leave you with a scene from one of my favorite movies, The Dead Poet's Society, starring Robin Williams who plays a high school teacher. He implores his students to, "seize the day and make your lives extraordinary." I implore you to seize the night, for only then will the day be yours. Verify your sleep ability and make sure you're living the best life possible.

Final Words from Dr. Mark Burhenne

Modern life has forced us to accept certain myths about our destiny. One of these myths is that our health will steadily deteriorate as we get older. One of my patients even told me his doctor said during his checkup, "It's all pretty much downhill from here, so you need to adjust your expectations."

But with uninterrupted sleep, it doesn't have to be that way! The healing powers of uninterrupted sleep actually square off this steady decline so that health stays good until the very end. This is called squaring the life curve, and it's a concept you don't find too often in modern medicine. It's not just about living longer—it's about the quality of your years.

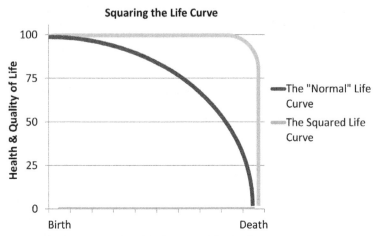

Instead of accepting health that steadily declines as we age, we can square the life curve by preventing illness and disease.

Taking charge of your sleep ability isn't easy, but you can do it.

My hope is that you'll take this book as your guide, follow its advice, and square your own life curve. Don't just read this book; use it. Share it with your sleep partner and other loved ones.

I also invite you to join our support group at *AsktheDentist. com/forum/sleep-apnea* which is a community of others who have read this book. I and other people in the community will be answering questions and providing support.

If this book helped you in any way, please share your thoughts with a review on Amazon or Goodreads. These reviews are essential to help other people find this information. A review is one of the best steps you can take to help get the word out. Let's get out this information together.

To your best breathing and great health,

Mark Burhenne, DDS

mark@askthedentist.com

Twitter: *@askthedentist*

P.S. I would love to hear from you. Write or tweet me with the first action step you plan to take after reading this book.

Acknowledgements

Any book about something as complicated as sleep-disordered breathing is never truly written by one person alone. This book would not exist without the countless hours that researchers, physicians, and scientists have given to understanding the complex world of sleep and the physiology of the airway.

Acknowledgements to my staff, for having such high standards in all that they do for our patients and for making it possible to do the work I love every day. Acknowledgements to my editors, Jeannie Ingraham and Deborah Natelson, for sharing their tremendous writing gifts, critical minds, and honest feedback. Part of the definition of doctor is "teacher"—a profession that depends on communication. I thank them for helping me better convey this important message.

I've been blogging about dental health since the mid-90s, but it wasn't until pioneers in health such as Dr. Ronesh Sinha, Dr. Alan Greene, Dr. Mark Hyman, Mark Sisson, Dr. Andrew Weil, Dr. Frank Lipman, Dr. Dean Ornish, Dr. Brian Palmer, Dr. Steven Park, and Dr. David Perlmutter came along that I really understood my role as a healthcare provider, which is: you don't just get the message out to a few people; you maximize the message by reaching as many people as possible. I remember reading Dean Ornish before I was a dental student and thinking to myself, *This is how medicine should be practiced.* Because of the Internet and the people who paved the way for me, I am privileged to be able to reach more people for the betterment of all of our health.

I must give my most sincere thanks to the American Academy of Dental Sleep Medicine. If it wasn't for their program, I would not be writing these words today. It is the education of the doctor that provides for great health care. The years I've spent with the AADSM have not only been inspirational, but they have also allowed me to better serve my patients. I am also grateful to my dental colleagues, namely Drs. Ariana and Max Ebrahimian who are leaders in the dental sleep medicine space.

You're not really a doctor unless you have patients who listen, right? I thank my patients for allowing me to treat them and for their enthusiasm and open-mindedness for something that they'd never heard of before, especially from their dentist. They have taught me more than they'll ever realize. I am also indebted to the countless people who have reminded me and encouraged me, saying, "Dr. Burhenne, you need to get this message out to the world."

I also am thankful to my family members, who have encouraged me, listened to me, and traveled to different cities to attend conferences with me. I have received nothing but encouragement and love from them throughout my training as a sleep medicine dentist and the writing of this book. Getting encouragement from people you care about is the best form of inspiration there is.

To my sister Yvonne, who has been instrumental in getting out not only this book but also the TEDx that goes along with it: you are my best critic, my most valued critic, and your support and feedback always mean so much. Thank you for the love and support.

To my daughters, to whom I'm grateful for explaining to me the importance of the web, the importance of blogging about the mouth-body connection and helping others through the internet, and for taking care of everything that goes on in the backend of AsktheDentist.com: there is no way I could answer questions online without you.

To my wife, Roseann, who so willingly was my first sleep apnea patient and my first great success in treating sleep apnea: thank you! The journey we've taken together has been more meaningful with you by my side. Watching you every day taking command of your health has shown me that it's possible to inspire others to do the same. I wake up every day grateful to be by your side.

Lastly, I thank my eldest daughter, Catharine: if it were not for her countless hours of editing and work on everything associated with this book and AsktheDentist.com, these words would not be here in print today. She has been a partner throughout the conception and execution of this book. It is for her and her generation that we worked—that they may start earlier with verifying their sleep ability and prevent the issues of their parents' generation; that they may go on to be the first generation of many to be healthier than their parents.

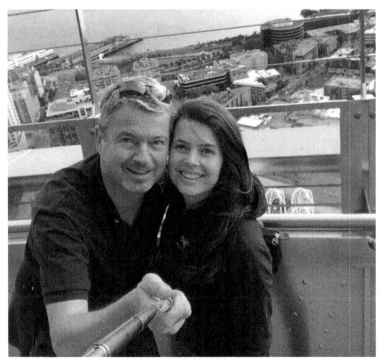

This is me and my eldest daughter, Catharine, who accompanied me to the American Academy of Dental Sleep Medicine conference in Seattle June of 2015 to assist with the creation of this book. We hope you enjoyed it!

Resources

Mark Burhenne, DDS

877 West Fremont Ave Suite E2

Sunnyvale, California 94087

www.markburhennedds.com

Ask the Dentist Email Newsletter

AsktheDentist.com is my own blog. Subscribe to the newsletter to get updates on the latest on sleep-disordered breathing and the mouth-body connection.

AsktheDentist.com/subscribe

The 8-Hour Sleep Paradox

Sleep Breathing Support Forum — Ask the Dentist

Join a community of others who have read this book. We will be answering questions and providing support.

AsktheDentist.com/forum/sleep-apnea

Brian Palmer, DDS

One of the original thinkers in the area of dental sleep medicine. This site is a great resource, although technical.

http://www.brianpalmerdds.com/Default.htm

Steven Park, MD

Dr. Park is an integrative ENT who is board certified in sleep medicine and runs a fantastic blog and podcast about the entire spectrum of sleep-disordered breathing.

www.doctorstevenpark.com

ClinicalTrials.gov

If you can't afford a sleep study, check out *http://www. clinicaltrials.gov*. You can search their database to find clinical studies in your local area that are recruiting people to participate in polysomnography sleep studies.

Find a Myofuncional Therapist in Your Area

http://www.myoacademy.net/myofunctional-therapist

Find a Dentist – American Academy of Dental Sleep Medicine

http://www.localsleepdentist.com

Find a Functional Medicine Practitioner – The Institute for Functional Medicine

https://www.functionalmedicine.org/practitioner_search. aspx?id=117

CPAP Assistance Program – Do you need a CPAP machine or know someone who does?

The American Sleep Apnea Association, through the CPAP Assistance Program (CAP) provides help for diagnosed sleep apnea patients who have no insurance, high insurance deductibles, or through financial hardship cannot afford this critical and life saving medical equipment.

http://www.sleepapnea.org/resources/cpap-assistance-program.html

A.W.A.K.E. Network – "Alert, Well, And Keeping Energetic"

Find a support group in the US or Canada via the American Sleep Apnea Association website's database of A.W.A.K.E. education and support groups.

http://www.sleepapnea.org/support/a.w.a.k.e.-network-map.html (Canada or the US)

If there isn't a support group in your area, email *awake@ sleepapnea.org*. Groups can be started by doctors or dentists, sleep technicians and sleep labs, hospitals and clinics, and patients volunteers- just to name a few.

CPAPTalk.com

There is a wealth of information on this site and tons of people who know exactly what you're going through and ready to provide answers and support. *CPAPTalk.com* is a community of over 31,000 registered members whose combined knowledge equals years and years of first hand sleep apnea experience, all in various stages of diagnosis and treatment, as well as their families, sleep doctors, sleep technicians, and equipment providers.

Insurance FAQ from the American Academy of Dental Sleep Medicine

http://www.aadsm.org/Resources/pdf/FAQInsuranceReimbursement.pdf

MAD Insurance Information, Including Codes

http://www.dentaleconomics.com/articles/print/volume-103/issue-5/features/you-can-do-it-oral-sleep-apnea-therapy-coded-correctly.html

MyPillow.com

Follow the instructions at *http://www.mypillow.com* to find a pillow that fits you to keep your spine straight and your airway tilted back if you sleep on your back. A pillow for side sleeping will be taller than a pillow for sleeping on your back so that your spine is kept in alignment. The pillows on this site are allergy-friendly and can thrown in the washer and dryer.

SnorLess Strips

SnorLess Strips are hypoallergenic, soft, don't hurt when you take them off, and won't leave marks on your face when mouth taping.

http://www.amazon.com/Snorless-Strips-Buteyko-Breathing-Method/dp/B002F915EO

The 8-Hour Sleep Paradox

SleepAnalyzer App (iOS) and Sleep Talk Recorder (Android)

These apps are quick and dirty tests to determine if you have disturbances in your sleep. They work by recording sounds throughout the night. When I test the SleepAnalyzer, I get between zero and 5 recordings when sleeping with my MAD and 250 to 450 recordings without the MAD (this has nothing to do with AHI and as we've discussed, cannot replace a polysomnography sleep study). I have not tested Sleep Talk Recorder since I don't have an Android device, but it works in the same way to record disturbances during the night.

Xlear Nasal Spray

This is a xylitol nasal spray designed to help open the nasal passageways without steroids or other drugs. You can use it continually without the rebound effects typical with other decongestants. Xylitol is a sugar that is antimicrobial and anti-inflammatory.

http://www.amazon.com/Xlear-Nasal-Spray-1-5-oz/dp/ B000M4W2E6

BMI Calculator – Mayo Clinic

BMI (Body Mass Index) is a measure of whether you're at a healthy weight. BMI is calculated as your weight (in kilograms) over your height squared (in centimeters). A healthy BMI ranges between 19 and 25. See the Mayo Clinic BMI Calculator to calculate your BMI: *http://www.mayoclinic.org/diseases-conditions/ obesity/in-depth/bmi-calculator/itt-20084938*

Appendix A:
Allergy-Proofing the Bedroom
for Serene Breathing

Even the most perfect, wide-open airway is susceptible to swelling from allergies. One of my patients, Dave, was thrilled when I told him he did not appear to be at risk for sleep-disordered breathing after a routine sleep-disordered breathing screening in the dental chair.

I turned around to change my gloves and grab a different mirror, and then I heard it. And then I heard it again. Dave was sniffling. I asked him if he had allergies. He replied that he constantly got sinus infections and had had asthma as a kid. He was struggling from hay fever after having to walk outside to the train station.

I asked Dave if he ever struggled to breathe through his nose. "No . . ." he responded. "Well, yeah, I guess whenever my allergies flare up."

I explained to Dave how even a wide-open airway doesn't mean you can't have sleep breathing difficulty at night, and that I suspected that his allergies, asthma, or both could be causing him trouble. I referred him to an allergist as well as an ENT to see if he had a blockage in his nose, such as a deviated septum.

Another one of my patients, Ciara, didn't seem to have any trouble breathing through her nose. She didn't exhibit any of the usual sleep-disordered breathing signs. I could tell by looking at her teeth that she wasn't grinding them. But there was one red flag. After I asked about the way she sniffled during her 7 a.m. appointment, she said, "Oh, the sniffles? Yeah, it's the weirdest thing. Lately, when I wake up in the morning, I'm stuffed up, but it always goes away right away. You're just seeing this since I woke up only fifteen minutes ago to come to this appointment."

As it turned out, Ciara's bedroom was not optimized for sleep breathing, and she was reacting to dust mites.

Dust mites avoid the light and need at least 50% relative humidity to survive. This is why they're so plentiful in soft materials like our pillows, mattresses, blankets, and bedsheets. Beds are their ideal environment: warm, dark, humid, and full of tasty skin scales.

A Better Bedroom for Better Breathing and Better Sleep

✓ Use allergen-impermeable covers for your pillows, mattress, and box spring to prevent mite allergens from escaping and being inhaled. You can also buy a pillow manufactured with an allergen barrier outer fabric.

✓ Wash all bedding every two weeks. This kills live mites and washes out mite allergen waste products. Hot water is best.

✓ Replace bed comforters with a special comforter manufactured with an allergen-barrier outer fabric. This won't need to be washed as frequently, since it cannot be colonized by mites.

✓ Remove bedroom carpet if you can in favor of a wipeable floor like hardwood, tile, or cement.

✓ Remove stuffed toys, throw pillows, pennants, upholstered furniture, and other non-washable, non-wipeable items from the bedroom. Make sure that special teddy bear is machine washed regularly.

✓ Use wipeable blinds or shades instead of curtains, or wash or dry-clean curtains frequently.

✓ If you can't remove carpet, use dry carpet-cleaning product to remove dust and mite allergens.

✓ Avoid shampooing the carpet, since the moisture can increase mite growth.

✓ Keep humidity below 50% to prevent dust mite growth entirely. Use A/C in the summer along with an additional dehumidifier.

✓ Avoid using a humidifier in the winter.

✓ Keep pets out of the bedroom. Let them sleep somewhere else in the house. Their dander can cause you to react.

✓ Use a HEPA air cleaner.

Appendix B:
Medicare-Approved Sleep
Apnea Appliances

As of January 4, 2013, these are the only devices that are eligible for Medicare reimbursement:[44]

- ✓ Herbst by Dynaflex
- ✓ Herbst by Gergen's Orthodontic Lab
- ✓ TAP by Airway Management
- ✓ TAP 3 Elite by Airway Management
- ✓ Telescopic Herbst by Great Lakes Orthodontics
- ✓ SUAD by Strong Dental LTD
- ✓ SUAD Elite by Strong Dental LTD
- ✓ UCLA Modified Herbst by Space Maintainers Laboratory

---

44   "Medicare PDAC Verifies More Devices," *American Academy of Dental Sleep Medicine*, 2013, *http://www.aadsm.org/articles.aspx?id=3565*.

Appendix C:
The ESS Questionnaire

How likely are you to doze off or fall asleep in the following situations, in contrast to feeling just tired? This refers to your usual way of life in recent times. Even if you have not done some of these things recently, try to work out how they would have affected you. Use the following scale to choose the most appropriate number for each situation:

0 = No chance of dozing

1 = Slight chance of dozing

2 = Moderate chance of dozing

3 = High chance of dozing

Epworth Sleepiness Scale (ESS)[45]

---

45   "Epworth Sleepiness Scale (ESS)," Inova, revised 09/25/08,*https://www.inova.org/upload/docs/Healthcare%20Services/Sleep%20Disorders/epworth-sleepiness-scale.pdf.*

Situation

(Chance of Dozing. Enter 0, 1, 2, 3, or 4)

___Sitting and reading

___Watching TV

___Sitting inactive in a public place (e.g. a theater or a meeting)

___As a passenger in a car for an hour without a break

___Lying down to rest in the afternoon when circumstances permit

___Sitting and talking to someone

___Sitting quietly after a lunch without alcohol

___In a car, while stopped for a few minutes in traffic

If you score a 9 or higher, you're more likely to get it covered by insurance and your primary care physician knows to recommend a sleep study for you.

1-6: Congratulations, you are getting enough sleep!

7-8: Your score is average.

9 and up: Seek the advice of a sleep specialist without delay.

Appendix D:
Data Points on the PSG to
Discuss With Your Doctor

Don't forget to get a copy of your PSG!

What a PSG Records:

- ✓ Brain wave activity (EEG)
- ✓ Eye movement (EOG)
- ✓ Muscle tone (measured with a chin strap)
- ✓ Airflow via thin catheters placed in the front of nostrils and mouth
- ✓ Breathing effort via belts placed over chest and abdomen
- ✓ Snoring (microphone over your neck)
- ✓ Heart rhythm (EKG)
- ✓ Oxygen level
- ✓ Leg muscle activity
- ✓ Body position
- ✓ Video recording

Number of Arousals

Each apneic event is referred to as an arousal.

Apnea Hypopnea Index (AHI)

The AHI is the frequency of breathing interruptions recorded during the study per hour of sleep. These interruptions can be apneas (temporary cessation of breathing) or hypopneas (abnormally slow or shallow breathing). AHI is generally expressed as the number of events per hour. An apnea is defined as 10 seconds or longer, so interruptions that are fewer than nine seconds are not counted—but still impact sleep and health.

Based on AHI, the severity of obstructive sleep apnea is classified as follows:

None/Minimal: AHI < 5 per hour (i.e. sleep interrupted fewer than 5 times per hour)

Mild: AHI ≥ 5, but < 15 per hour (i.e. sleep interrupted 5-14 times per hour)

Moderate: AHI ≥ 15, but < 30 per hour (i.e. sleep interrupted 15-29 times per hour)

Severe: AHI ≥ 30 per hour (i.e. sleep interrupted at least 30 times per hour)

Ideally, of course, one should measure not just every time breathing is interrupted but also every time breathing is made difficult—such as by partial blockages. But the AHI is still a good start.

Respiratory Disturbance Index (RDI)

Sometimes, the Respiratory Disturbance Index (RDI) is used to measure results. This can be confusing, because the RDI includes not only apneas and hypopneas but also other, more subtle breathing irregularities. This means that your RDI can be higher than your AHI.

Oxygen Desaturation

The PSG will measure how much the oxygen level in the blood decreases. At sea level, a normal blood oxygen level (saturation) is usually 96 to 97%. Although there are no generally accepted classifications for severity of oxygen desaturation, reductions down to 90% usually are considered mild. Dips into the 80 to 89% range can be considered moderate, and those below 80% are severe.[46]

Non-Airway Factors That Impact Your PSG Results

Looking at your health history can shed some light on what you might see during your sleep study. For example, various medications can alter how long it takes for you to go to sleep (sleep latency), your AHI, and how much oxygen gets to your brain. For this reason, I strongly recommend having your health history at your fingertips when seeing your sleep doctor.

---

46   "Understanding the Results." *Apnea*. Division of Sleep Medicine at Harvard Medical School, 2011, *http://healthysleep.med.harvard.edu/sleep-apnea/diagnosing-osa/understanding-results.*

Questions to Ask Your Doctor

✓ *Did I have any central apneas (i.e. apneas caused by the brain not sending out the right signals)? How many?*

✓ *Did I breathe or leak through my mouth? How often? What do you recommend to prevent it?*

✓ *Can I take care of this without getting surgery? If you recommend surgery, what is the drawback to trying a non-surgical technique to see if that works first, like CPAP or oral appliance therapy?*

✓ *Did I exhibit positional sleep apnea? Was my apnea more severe in one sleeping position than in others? Is my pressure requirement higher in one position than others?*

✓ *Is there anything else unusual about the results?*

✓ *How will I know my therapy is preventing apneas?*

✓ *I would like to own a data-capable machine and software to monitor apneas, hypopneas, and mask leak. Will you help me with the appropriate prescription?*

✓ *How will I know if and when I've cured my sleep apnea?*

✓ *Can I achieve an AHI of zero? (The answer is, yes, you can! And that should be the goal!)*

Sleep-disordered breathing can be broken down into three categories:

✓ **Obstructive:** Breathing is being interrupted or slowed by a physical obstruction.

✓ **Central:** This is when the brain fails to send a signal to tell the body to breathe.

✓ **Mixed:** A mix of both obstructive and central.

Appendix E:
Factors Other Than the Epworth (ESS) to Determine Whether You Get a PSG (Attended Sleep Study)

Review this list and inform your doctor if you have any of the following:

✓ Stroke

✓ High blood pressure

✓ Heart disease

✓ Family history of sleep apnea

✓ Bed partner or sleep app reported snoring, gasping/choking, stop breathing at night

✓ Daytime sleepiness or tiredness

✓ Drowsy driving

✓ GERD (gastroesophageal reflux disease)

✓ Morning headaches, dry mouth, sore throat

✓ Decreased sex drive

✓ Waking up to go to the bathroom in the middle of the night

✓ Mood, memory, or attention problems

✓ Twitching and jerking limbs at night

✓ Difficulty falling or staying asleep

✓ Falling asleep right when you hit the pillow (under five minutes)

✓ Gout[47]

STOP-BANG Sleep Apnea Questionnaire:[48]

Tally up the number of times you answered "yes." This is your score.

5 - 8: High risk of obstructive sleep apnea

3 - 4: Intermediate risk of obstructive sleep apnea

0 - 2: Low risk of obstructive sleep apnea

---

47   http://www.ncbi.nlm.nih.gov/pmc/articles/PMC2654829/

48   F. Chung et al, "STOP-BANG Sleep Apnea Questionnaire,"Anesthesiology (2008) and BJA (2012). Ohio Sleep Medicine Institute, accessed 10/2015, https://www.sleepmedi-cine.com/files/files/StopBang_Questionnaire.pdf.

The STOP-BANG Questionnaire

STOP		
Do you **S**NORE loudly (louder than talking or loud enough to be heard through closed doors)?	Yes	No
Do you often feed **T**IRED, fatigued, or sleepy during daytime?	Yes	No
Has anyone **O**BSERVED you stop breathing during your sleep?	Yes	No
Do you have or are you being treated for high blood **P**RESSURE?	Yes	No

BANG		
BMI (Body Mass Index) greater than 35?	Yes	No
AGE over 50 years old?	Yes	No
NECK circumference greater than 16 inches (40 cm)?	Yes	No
GENDER: Male?	Yes	No

Appendix F:
Myofunctional Therapy Exercises for
Sleep-Disordered Breathing
By Sarah Hornsby, RDH, Myofunctional Therapist,
www.myfaceology.com

Step One:

Learn to breathe through your nose all day, with your mouth closed.

If you already do this, then you're one step ahead. If you don't, a good way to start learning to breathe through your nose is by setting a timer.

I recommend placing a piece of tape gently across your lips, starting with just five or ten minutes at a time. Add five minutes every few days until you can work up to one hour with tape across your lips. Practice once a day, until it feels natural to breathe through your nose for longer periods of time.

Step Two:

Learn where to rest your tongue inside your mouth.

The area where the tip of your tongue should rest is called the "Spot." When your mouth is closed, and you are breathing through your nose, this is where your tongue should always rest.

You can find the Spot by starting with the tip of your tongue touching the backside of your upper front teeth. Move your tongue slightly backwards until you feel a bumpy ridge area and a small depression. This position is a little different for everyone, but in general, the Spot should be located about a quarter of an inch directly behind your upper front teeth, on the roof of your mouth.

Practice timing yourself with your tongue on the Spot, just like in the first exercise. Start with five minutes at a time, and slowly work up to one hour each day, until it becomes more natural for your tongue to rest on the Spot.

Step Three:

Use exercises to strengthen the muscles in your tongue, lips, cheeks, and throat. Below are eleven exercises that I recommend practicing twice every day. It takes about 10 minutes to go through all of them in a row.

1. Tongue brushing
2. Suction and hold
3. Tongue trace
4. Left, right, up, down
5. Jaw resistance
6. Forcing air
7. Yawn pulls
8. Ahhh sounds
9. Eee ooo aaaa
10. Finger in cheek
11. Reach for the ceiling (bonus: add swallow)

Tongue Brushing

1. Using your toothbrush, brush the top and sides of your tongue.

2. Keep your tongue in the floor of your mouth, or stretched outside of your mouth about half way.

3. Brush the following sections of your tongue each times each.

   a. Left side

   b. Top (down the center)

   c. Right side

   d. Tip

4. Repeat this cycle three times.

Suction and Hold

1. Start by making a "click" with your tongue. This will demonstrate the feeling of your tongue being suctioned to the roof of your mouth.

2. Next, try sticking your tongue to the roof of our mouth without letting it unstick to make a clicking sound.

3. Once your tongue is "suctioned" to the roof of your mouth, open wide, and bring your cheeks back into a smiling position.

4. Hold this position for 10 seconds, then rest for 2 seconds.

5. Repeat 6 times.

Tongue Trace

1. Start with your mouth open about halfway, and your cheeks back in a smiling position.

2. Slide the tip of your tongue from the backside of your upper front teeth, along your palate towards the back of your throat.

3. Repeat 20 times.

Left, Right, Up, Down

1. Open your mouth wide.

2. Stick your tongue out as far as it will go, out the left side of your mouth.

3. Count to 10.

4. Repeat this for the right side of your mouth, then up towards your nose, and lastly, down towards your chin. Hold each position for 10 seconds as well.

5. Repeat the whole cycle (Left, Right, Up Down) three times.

Jaw Resistance

1. Place your hand underneath your chin.

2. Attempt to open your mouth while using your hand to push against your chin, creating a resistance.

3. Hold for 5 seconds, then rest for 2 seconds.

4. Repeat 10 times.

Forcing Air

1. Take a deep breath, and purse your lips together.

2. Exhale, and using your diaphragm and abdomen, force the air out from between your pursed lips. This should feel similar to blowing up a balloon.

3. Force the air out for 5 seconds.

4. Repeat 10 times.

Yawn Pulls

1. Looking in a mirror, open your mouth wide, and find your uvula. This is the area in the back of your throat that hangs down to form a ball or oblong shape.

2. Watching your uvula, try to make yourself yawn by raising that part of your throat upwards. If you can't yawn, that's okay, just focus on the movement instead.

3. Hold this position for 5 seconds, then rest for 2 seconds.

4. Repeat 10 times.

Ahhh Sounds

1. Looking in a mirror, start with your mouth open wide, and your tongue inside of your mouth.

2. Make an "ahhh" sound for 5 seconds, while pushing your tongue downward, towards the floor of your mouth at the same time.

3. Repeat this 8 times.

The 8-Hour Sleep Paradox

Eee Ooo Aaa

1. Start by moving your cheeks back to form a big smile. You can say the "eee" sound out loud, or do this silently.. The goal is to use large, over-exaggerated movements so that your facial muscles have to work hard.

2. Hold the "eee" position for 10 seconds.

3. Repeat this with the position used to say "oooh", and then the position used to say "ahhh". Remember to use exaggerated movements.

4. Repeat the "eee-ooo-aaa" cycle three times.

Finger in Cheek

1. Open your mouth about halfway, and place your first finger inside your cheek.

2. Push your finger so it moves your cheek outwards.

3. Contract your cheek and lips, so that the muscles resist the pushing.

4. Repeat 10 times for each cheek.

Reach for the Ceiling

1. Tilt your head back so that you are looking at the ceiling.

2. Stick your tongue out as if you are attempting to touch the ceiling with it.

3. Hold this position for 10 seconds.

4. Repeat 5 times.

5. Bonus: To make this exercise even more challenging, you can try to gently bite your tongue and swallow in this position.

Appendix G:
Insurance Form For When You Can't Tolerate a CPAP

Affidavit of Intolerance to CPAP

(Continuous Positive Air Pressure)

I have attempted to use nasal CPAP to manage my sleep disordered breathing (obstructive sleep apnea) and find it intolerable to use on a regular basis due to the following reason(s):

- ❑ PAP is not effective in controlling my symptoms.
- ❑ I am unable to sleep with the CPAP equipment in place.
- ❑ Noise from the device disturbs my sleep or my bed partner's sleep.
- ❑ I cannot find a comfortable mask.
- ❑ The mask leaks.
- ❑ I develop sinus / throat / ear / lung infections.
- ❑ I am allergic to materials in the mask and head straps.
- ❑ Claustrophobia.
- ❑ I unconsciously remove the CPAP apparatus at night.
- ❑ Pressure from the mask and straps causes tissue breakdown.

❏ My job and/or lifestyle prevents this form of therapy (e.g. Active Army / National Guard duty).

❏ Prior throat surgery makes CPAP intolerable.

❏ Other: _____

Because of my inability to tolerate CPAP and my need to control the signs and symptoms of OSA, I wish to use an alternative method of treatment. This form of therapy is a mandibular advancement device (MAD).

Signed: _____ Date: _____

Also By Mark Burhenne, DDS

SLEEPYHEAD
How Your Child's Oral Development Determines
How They Sleep for the Rest of Their Lives

Available 2017

Sign up at *AsktheDentist.com/sleepyhead* for a free chapter.

There is more knowledge than ever about how to raise a healthy child, and yet our children are suffering from chronic health conditions and behavioral disorders at rates never seen before. The missing link? Sleep ability, which Dr. Burhenne describes as the body's ability to breathe easily even in the deepest stages of sleep.

According to Dr. Burhenne, this health epidemic isn't about getting enough sleep—rather, getting the right kind of sleep. A child who grows up with the modern diet and lifestyle has an airway that is much narrower from those of children 100 years ago. Understanding how a child's face, jaw, and airway grow is essential to ensuring optimal sleep for a lifetime—and it's all set in stone by the time a child is 10 years old.

Informed by cutting-edge science and a new paradigm for considering the epigenetics of oral development, along with case studies from children who have experienced life-changing transformations, *Sleepyhead* is an illuminating look at the hidden cause behind what is making our children sick and an action plan to ensure your child develops well and thrives with the sleep they deserve.

Made in the USA
Las Vegas, NV
23 November 2022

60083058R00105